PUBLICATIONS OF
THE WELLCOME INSTITUTE OF THE
HISTORY OF MEDICINE

General Editor: F. N. L. Poynter, Ph.D., D.Litt., Hon. M.D. (Kiel)

New Series, Volume XVII

ROBERT WHYTT,
THE SOUL, AND MEDICINE

by R. K. French

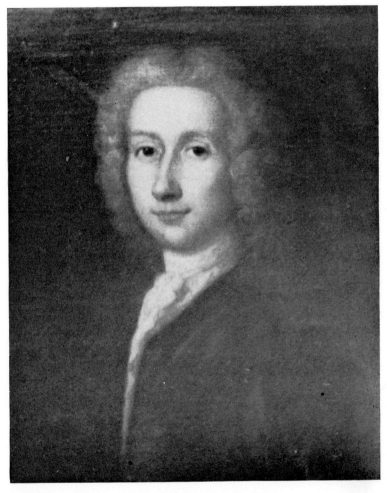

ROBERT WHYTT (1714-1766)
The Bellucci portrait, formerly in the possession of the late
E. W. M. Balfour Melville

ROBERT WHYTT, THE SOUL, AND MEDICINE

by

R. K. French

London
THE WELLCOME INSTITUTE OF THE
HISTORY OF MEDICINE
1969

© R. K. French, 1969

Made and printed in Great Britain
at the St Ann's Press, Park Road, Altrincham

Acknowledgments

My thanks are due to Dr. A. C. Crombie of Oxford University, who first suggested Robert Whytt as a subject for research, and to Dr. W. H. Brock, Dr. K. D. Keele and Dr. F. N. L. Poynter, whose constructive criticism enabled me to turn the resultant thesis into what I hope is a readable book.

R.K.F.

Contents

Robert Whytt (1714–1766): The Bellucci portrait, formerly
in the possession of the late E. W. M. Balfour Melville.

CHAPTER I

The Life of Robert Whytt

Witta, whose last resting place lies close upon Edinburgh, shares
the distinction of being a great-grandfather of Hengist and Horsa,
according to legend,[1] with that of being a more distant forebear of
Robert Whytt. More cautious judgements[2] give the family a
French origin, but speculation only ceases with Matthew Whyte of
Maw, who was granted a charter in 1492. Matthew's descendants
became wealthy landowners of increasing influence in Fife, inter-
marrying with the better-known families of Melville (whose name
Robert Whytt's son was to adopt) and Balfour, who were to provide
Robert's second wife.

Robert's great-grandfather was another Robert, who added to
his own wealth that of the heiress he married. He became first
Provost of Kirkcaldy, and was in 1647 appointed Member of the
Committee of Estates by Parliament. He was known as the Baron
of Bennochy, but the title[3] refers not to a peerage[4] but to his powers
of 'pit and gallows'[5] as a landlord. His son John married Jean
Melville and was the father of a second Robert, who was 'bred in
law' and admitted to the Faculty of Advocates in 1694. Relating
to him are a large number of legal documents in the family's
possession; his own contract of marriage to Jean Murray, 'a woman

---

[1] W. Seller, 'Memoir of the life and writings of Robert Whytt, M.D., Professor
of Medicine in the University of Edinburgh, 1714-1766', *Trans. R. Soc. Edinb.*,
1862, 23, 99.

[2] Sir Robert Douglas, *History of the Baronage of Scotland*, Edinburgh, 1798.
The arms resemble those of the Les Blancs: Argent, a martlet displayed between
three-quarter foils sable; on a chief of the last, as many quarter-foils of the first.
Crest: dexter hand, couped at the shoulder, holding a wreath of laurel proper.
Motto: *Virtute Parta*. The name is properly pronounced 'white', and Robert was
unusual in adopting the spelling 'Whytt' rather than 'Whyte'.

[3] Sir Robert Douglas, op. cit.

[4] W. Anderson, *Scottish Nation*, Edinburgh, 1863, vol. 3, p. 637. There is also a
reference to the 'barony' in the papers of E. W. M. Balfour Melville, a descendant
of Robert Whytt, for whose help in the early stages of this work I am grateful.
After his death his papers were moved to the Scottish Record Office.

[5] B. Balfour Melville, *The Balfours of Pilrig*, Edinburgh, 1907, p. 135. In J. Brown,
The Epitaphs and Monumental Inscriptions in Greyfriars Churchyard, Edinburgh, 1867,
Robert Whytt is described as a knight. This is a mistranslation of *armiger*.

not less remarkable by her manner than her rank', daughter of Anthony Murray of Woodend, in Perthshire, is dated 16 February 1697.[6] He had the reputation of being an intelligent lawyer and honest man, but he died on 23 February 1714, six months before the birth of his second son, Robert. The eldest son was George.

Robert Whytt was born in Edinburgh on 10 September 1714. Shortly after his birth, his widowed mother left Edinburgh for Kirkcaldy. Bower was 'not informed who had charge of his early education',[7] but Barclay,[8] from an unpublished and undated Harveian Oration in the possession of Mrs. Balfour Melville, says that Robert at the public school af Kirkcaldy, 'soon exhibited the conspicuous and decisive marks of uncommon superiority of talents'.

In 1717 his brother George matriculated at St. Andrews. His college was St. Salvator's, then, according to Defoe,[9] 'in its declining state and looking into its grave'. However, the records of the period are good and 'Georgius Whytt de Bennochy'[10] appears in his hand on the register. He began his studies as a second-year student and left without taking a degree. This was not uncommon but in George's case may have been owing to the death of his mother in, or about, 1720. He was, however, granted an M.A. and M.D. on 13 June 1726, probably, as there is no signature, in his absence. According to the inventory mentioned below (see appendix) George also received a diploma three days later. In 1728, having 'given proofs of spirit and abilities which excited in his friends the highest expectations',[11] he died, and Robert, who had been in his care, came into the estate.

Most authorities agree that Robert Whytt entered St. Andrews University about 1727, but, in fact, this seems open to doubt. The usual sources are Seller and Bower, who do not give references, and the euphonius commonplaces of the Harveian Oration give no hint of originality. The records of St. Andrews, which bear witness to George Whytt's matriculation and degrees, offer no confirmation of Robert's entry in 1727 or any M.A. of 1730. The latter date

[6] According to a list of members of the Faculty of Advocates, compiled by the Scottish Record Society, the date of the actual marriage was 14 February.

[7] A. Bower, *History of the University of Edinburgh*, Edinburgh, 1817, p. 350.

[8] All quotations from the Harveian Oration are taken from R. Mary Barclay, *The Life and Work of Robert Whytt: A Preliminary Survey*, (part of an M.D. thesis) Edinburgh, 1922.

[9] G. S. Pryde, *Scotland from 1603 to the Present Day*, (vol. 2 of *A New History of Scotland*), Edinburgh, 1962, p. 108.

[10] I am indebted to the Keeper of the Muniments of the University of St. Andrews for extracts from the register.

[11] Harveian Oration.

2

given in Grant[12] and probably taken from Seller, is generally used to estimate the year of his matriculation. Several points argue against these dates and against St. Andrews: the absence of Whytt's name from the register, the fact that the normal course was four years, which would involve Whytt matriculating in 1726 at the age of twelve (most students being thirteen or fourteen), and the omission of any reference to the M.A. by the University authorities—or in his own supporting testimonials—when Whytt was awarded the M.D. degree.[13]

The records of Edinburgh University, on the other hand, show that a Robert Whyt matriculated in 1729. From 6 February until the end of the academic year he read philosophy under Professor Colin Drummond. It is known that Whytt began to study medicine at Edinburgh in 1730 and the records show us a Robert White in a class-list of Alexander Monro (*primus*) in 1731-2 and 1734,[14] whom we must identify with Whytt. It would be a great coincidence if the Whyt who finished his philosophy course in 1729 were not the same White who began his medical education in 1730. It is impossible to reconcile this with the four years Whytt would have needed to proceed to the degree of M.A. at St. Andrews. and it is likely that some confusion has arisen, either with another student, or with the degree of M.D. which he was given by St. Andrews several years later, particularly as the date of this second degree is always wrongly given; the few biographical accounts there are seem to depend on the same source, which is not entirely trustworthy.[15]

Monro and his fellow professors, Rutherford, Sinclair, Plummer, Alston and Innes, were then leading the Medical School at Edinburgh from its infancy to wide recognition. These were Whytt's teachers, and he had the satisfaction later of counting them among his colleagues. For Whytt, as for most of his fellow students (who included Fothergill, Armstrong and Eikenstein) no single medical school was a complete education, and in 1734 he left Edinburgh for London, bearing with him a recommendation from Monro to Cheselden, whose pupil he became.

For two years he gained experience in the wards of the London hospitals (no doubt at times a spectator of Cheselden's famous

[12] Sir Alexander Grant, *The Story of the University of Edinburgh during its First Three Hundred Years*, London, 1884, vol. 2, p. 401.

[13] My thanks are again due to the Keeper of the Muniments of St. Andrews for these interesting facts.

[14] For this I am indebted to the Matriculation Office and the Department of Manuscripts of the University of Edinburgh.

[15] We must also assume that several copies of legal documents (see appendix) which afford Whytt the premature title 'Doctor', although dated 1732, are retrospective errors.

swift lithotomies) and completed the greater part of his medical education. The finishing touches he acquired in Paris, visiting the wards of La Charité and L'Hôtel Dieu, hearing some of Winslow's lectures and others in L'Ecole de Médecine, and then in Leyden from the lectures of Albinus and the ageing Boerhaave.

This occupied but little time, for on 2 April 1736, he took his M.D. at Rheims. Perhaps he was moved to do so by a Scottish prudence in financial matters, for to have remained at Leyden and taken the degree there would have cost him sixteen pounds, 'apart from feasting the faculty',[16] an unusually expensive procedure. At all events he was not alone in this practice, for a third of the forty-eight new Fellows of the Edinburgh College of Physicians between 1700 and 1737 had Rheims degrees.

On his return to Scotland, the University of St. Andrews awarded Whytt an M.D. The date of this degree, given 'in eundem', appears on the records as 31 October 1737. All the biographical accounts give 3 June of the same year, a mistake which arises from confusion with another physician returning from Rheims and granted an M.D. 'in eundem' at St. Andrews. On 21 June he became a Licentiate of the Royal College of Physicians, Edinburgh, and on 27 November of the following year he was elected to the Fellowship and began to practise.

Accounts of the early days of his practice do not agree. Seller, probably from Bower, says his practice was extensive. Bower adds: 'to which no doubt he was considerably indebted to his old family connections, and being known to be in easy circumstances, but his own merit and the acknowledged superiority of his talents were principally what adduced to bring him into notice.'[17]

On the other hand the Harveian Oration says: 'although his abilities were universally allowed to be great, for several years his practice was not extensive, which is hardly to be wondered at when it is considered that so many practitioners of mature experience were in residence in Edinburgh.'

With or without an extensive practice, Whytt found time to get married. His bride was Helen Robertson,[18] sister of General

[16] J. Ruhräh, 'Robert Whytt, M.D., Professor of Medicine in the University of Edinburgh, 1714-66', *Journal of the Alumni Association of the College of Physicians and Surgeons Baltimore, Md.*, 1911, p. 74.

[17] A. Bower, op. cit., p. 350.

[18] According to Barbara Balfour-Melville, her name was Margaret. Quite inexplicable is the following extract from a letter written by Miss Betty Hamilton in 1842: 'Dr. Whytte was married before he married my aunt to a Mrs. Melville, a widow, by which he became stepfather to another family of Melvilles of some note in Fife. He was nearly related to the Whyttes of Kirkcaldie and to Miss Martha Whytte the heiress, afterwards Countess of Elgin . . .'. From B. Balfour-Melville, op. cit., p. 255.

4

Robertson, Governor of New York, but the date is apparently undiscoverable, being absent from the biographies and the registers of the three parishes of Edinburgh. They had two sons, both of whom died in infancy. It is no small tribute to Whytt that though his private life was full of tragedy, he was able to give constructive attention to the medical problems of his time. His parents' and his brother's early deaths and those of his first two children were soon followed by the untimely decease of his wife and of no less than eight of the children of his subsequent marriage. Yet during this time he was busy constructing and developing those ideas which here established his place in the history of medicine.

Thus in 1739 he began to question the contemporary accounts of the motion of the heart, of respiration, and the vital and involuntary motions generally, most of which accounts owed their standing to his teacher, Boerhaave. At the same time he became interested in discovering a medicine with which he could treat the stone of the bladder. Perhaps his interest sprang from his association with Cheselden, but it is more likely to have been aroused by the decision of Parliament to buy a secret remedy from Mrs. Joanna Stephens (for £5000) for the benefit of the poor. If the later observer is occasionally tempted to think that eighteenth-century gentlemen suffered from little else but gout and stone, no doubt those same gentlemen were often of a like opinion; there was, at all events, a great public interest in the malady, not a little heightened by the death of Sir Robert Walpole (Earl of Orford) which had been hastened by a lime-containing medicine for the stone. Doctors Ranby and Jurin, and Sir Edward Hulse became involved in a controversy which emphasized the dilemma facing the sufferer: whether to face the rigours and dangers of lithotomy or the lesser dangers, protracted unpleasantness and eventual uncertainty of a course of medicines.

Mrs. Stephens' medicine (published in June 1739 in the *London Gazette*) consisted of calcined egg shells, soap and aromatic bitters and not surprisingly was considered to be exceedingly unpleasant to take. The physicians of the country at once set to work to improve its taste and effectiveness. Whytt was among the first to isolate its 'active ingredient'—lime-water—and prepare it in a more palatable form. His evident success (however difficult it is to explain the action of lime-water in modern terms) was such that Sir Robert Walpole's brother Horace was eventually induced to attempt a cure and to furnish a number of letters of recommendation which were later incorporated in the *Works* of 1768.

Whytt embodied his ideas in a paper for the *Edinburgh Medical*

5

Essays of 1743.[19] It attracted a great deal of attention, and was the founding stone of his contemporary reputation. It was published separately and ran through several editions. The augmented version of 1752 was called *An Essay on the Virtues of Lime-Water in the Cure of the Stone*, which appeared again in Edinburgh in 1755 and in Dublin in 1762. In 1766 it was translated into French by Roux and appeared with Butter's account of dissolving the stone by injections. It was also translated into German by Kapp in 1771.[20]

His wife died in 1741.[21] Two years later, on 24 April 1743, he married Louisa Balfour, the daughter of James Balfour of Pilrig, and sister to a future professor of Moral Philosophy at Edinburgh. Louisa was known as the 'White Rose of Pilrig' and generally owned to be very beautiful. Her husband 'remained her lover until her death'[22] and she bore him fourteen children, of whom four died at about the age of a year and four at five years. Two sons survived their parents, but the male line was not carried further than one more generation.

The close association which had existed for generations between the Whytt and Melville families comes to light again with the entry of one Elizabeth Buchanan into the Maiden Hospital in 1740. The Maiden Hospital was dependent upon the Company of Merchants of the City of Edinburgh, and Mary Erskine, upon the funds of Mrs. Melville, widow of Doctor Andrew Melville. Lt. Robert Melville had the right of presentation of patients into the hospital, which, when he was abroad, was delegated to the care of Robert Whytt, along with 'managing his whole business and affaires'. A dissertation that Elizabeth Buchanan should be 'educate, entertained and provided for' was presented by Whytt from 1740 until at least 1748.[23]

An even closer connection appears in 1745, the year of rebellion, when perhaps Melville expected to see active service, for he asked

[19] 'An essay towards the discovery of a safe medicine for dissolving the stone', *Edinburgh Medical Essays*, 1743, 5, part 2. When the Medical Society became the Philosophical Society, its journal lost its title *Medical Essays and Observations* (usually known as the *Edinburgh Medical Essays*) and became *Essays and Observations, Physical and Literary* (known as *Edinburgh Essays, Physical and Literary*). This has given rise to some confusion.
[20] *Sämmtliche zur practischen Arzneykunst gehörige Schriften. Aus dem Englischen nach der neusten Ausgabe übersetzt*, Leipzig, 1771.
[21] The date is not given in the biographical sketches, but appears in the Greyfriars' Parish Register as 26 January. I am indebted for this information to the office of the Registrar-General.
[22] R. M. Barclay, op. cit.
[23] The dissertation is among the papers of E. W. M. Balfour-Melville, now in the Scottish Record Office.

Whytt to act as a 'commissioner' on his behalf, 'for managing his whole business and affaires within the kingdom of Scotland the same may be in the same manner as he could do himself if personally present'.[24]

By now Whytt had begun to formulate the physiological ideas that had occupied his mind for some years. His doctrine of the central part played by the 'sentient principle' in vital and involuntary motions was first expressed in a paper, the first of his later *Physiological Essays*, 'An Enquiry into the Causes which Promote the Circulation of Fluids in the Small Vessels of Animals'. This was read before the Philosophical Society of Edinburgh in 1745 or 1746 and no doubt served to draw further attention to the young physician already well known for his treatment of the stone with lime-water. By this or by his increasing practice, Whytt (now living in Blackfriars Wynd[25]) came to the attention of the Town Council, largely through whose efforts the Medical School of Edinburgh had been recently founded within the 'Town's College'. The 1745 rebellion may have caused a disturbance even within academic life, for a confusion exists over the date of Whytt's election as Professor of Medicine. The Harveian Oration says that when Sinclair found himself in failing health, he resigned his academic appointments in favour of Dr. Whytt; and that the latter's admission into College took place on 20 June 1746, 'and he began his first course in the Institutions of Medicine at the commencement of the next winter session'. Dezeimeris[26] also gives the date as 1746. Bower, Seller and later accounts give the date as 26 August 1747, taken from the 'Commission appointing him Professor of the Theory of Medicine'. As Bower adds that he had taught for some time in the college before his election, supplying the place of Innes, it may well be that the date of June 1746 refers to the start of Whytt's actual teaching, and it may be that it was during this time when Whytt 'gave universal content to all Gentlemen learned in that science', that the Register of Council recorded his election.

Clearly there was a great deal of informality about the early days of the Edinburgh Medical School; lectures were sometimes planned and not given, and the transition of a private physician to a college teacher could have been accomplished in stages. The first Monro gave anatomical lectures from 1720, but it is more

[24] Also in the Scottish Record Office. The commission is dated 25 March 1745, and registered in the books of Council of Session on 11 April.

[25] Now Blackfriars Street.

[26] J. Dezeimeris, *Dictionnaire historique de la Médecine ancienne et moderne*, Paris, 1839, vol. 4, p. 404.

just to regard the appointment by the Town Council of four Fellows of the Royal College of Physicians as the inception of the Medical School. These four were Rutherford, Plummer, Sinclair and Innes. Two years earlier, indeed, Porterfield had been appointed Professor of the Institutes and the Practice of Medicine, but it is not certain that he ever gave lectures. In 1730 the Senatus Academicus recognized five professors as a Medical Faculty. Rutherford and Innes lectured on the Practice of Medicine, Plummer on Chemistry, or rather Chemical Pharmacy, and Sinclair on the Theory of Medicine. After 1738 Alston lectured on Materia Medica and Botany.

In 1743 or 1744 Innes became ill and unable to continue with his duties. It was largely the vacancy in the four original professorships caused by the death of Innes which prompted the election of Whytt. Innes, however, was a supernumary professor, and Seller says that the real intention was that Whytt should fill Sinclair's duties. This seems to be borne out by the Harveian Oration which describes Whytt as lecturing in the Institutions of Medicine. Other sources say he was elected as Professor of the Theory of Medicine, but Bower says he was also Professor of the Practice of Medicine. It is likely that at first his duties were not rigidly determined, and that he might teach in all branches of medicine; it seems to have been stipulated on his appointment that even if another vacancy should occur, no new election should be held. Provost Drummond was instrumental in placing Whytt in the chair, and in seeking the consent of the Duke of Argyll, through his delegate, Lord Milton. These are doubtless the 'Patrons of the University' of the Harveian Oration, whose consent, with the 'approbation of the Medical Practitioners of Edinburgh, and the unanimous voice of the Publick' applauded Whytt's succession.

As professor, Whytt seems to have enlarged the reputation which 'carried him to the Chair'. He was noted for the accuracy and the elegance of the Latin of his lectures: the *Biographie Universelle*[27] speaks of his 'Latin plein d'élégance et de clarité', but his writings were all in English, possibly because he wanted them to have a wider audience—certainly his work on lime-water and nervous diseases were intended to be of immediate practical use. During these early years of his professorship, Whytt, preparing his first large work, remained active in the practical and academic spheres. There is in existence his eighth dissertation for the entry of Elizabeth Buchanan to the Maiden Hospital in 1748 and a testimonial, dated 1750, in support of a candidate for the St. Andrews M.D. degree

27 *Biographie Universelle*, Paris, 1827, vol. 44, p. 555.

In 1754 he published, in *Edinburgh Essays, Physical and Literary*, an essay 'Of the various Strengths of the different lime-waters'. This was occasioned by Dr. Alston's objections to Whytt's earliest ideas on lime-water.

During this time his teaching largely followed Boerhaave, and it was not until 1762 that he adopted instead the *Institutiones Pathologiae* of Gaub, Boerhaave's successor. His reservations upon certain of Boerhaave's ideas, and upon the general theories of the motion of the heart, and respiration were made clear when he published in 1751 his *Essay on the Vital and other Involuntary Motions of Animals*.[28] This must be regarded as his most important work. It sets out his scheme of physiology in full and shows clearly the part he considered that the soul, or 'sentient principle' played in animal motions. This separates his conceptions at once from the current 'mechanical' hypotheses and from the quite different animism of Stahl. In the book are to be found those contributions to neurophysiology which have drawn attention to him as an originator of the idea of reflex action.

The book was widely read and commented upon on the Continent as in Britain. Perhaps Whytt's European reputation (which was not inconsiderable) was furthered by the controversy he entered upon with Haller, who had criticized Whytt's book in a Göttingen book-review. 'Nothing', he had said, 'is more specious than to derive all motions from the soul'.[29] Whytt was lacking in candour and in imitating the asperity of the Stahlians, was more critical than constructive. Haller maintained that Whytt was a Stahlian in a later bibliographical compilation, noting in his favour only his 'great ingenuity'[30].

Nearer home, the *Essay* had a more favourable reception. The *Monthly Review* of March 1752, observed that it was a book

. . . which cannot fail, in the whole, of entertaining our medical and physiological readers. Besides the advantage of an appropriate and extensive erudition, which manifests itself without affectation or pedantry, our Author discovers a great natural fund of thinking. His conceptions are happy; his reasoning clear and strong; his expressions elegant, free, to the best of our recollection, from the least peculiarity of the Scottish idiom; and so adapted to his subject that it seems to flow of course from his intimate consideration of it.[31]

With his increasing fame, we have evidence of Whytt's wide

[28] Published in Edinburgh. There was a second edition in 1763.
[29] *Relationes de Novis Libris*, 1752, no. 1, part 3, p. 157.
[30] A. von Haller, *Bibliotheca Anatomica*, Zurich, 1774-77, vol. 2, p. 466.
[31] *Monthly Review*, 1752, *6*, 182, 449.

range of interests and correspondents. The eulogistic Harveian Oration asserts that 'His opinion on medical subjects was daily requested by Medical Authorities in every part of Britain' and that 'Foreigners of the first distinction and celebrated physicians of the most remote parts of the British Empire courted an intercourse with him by letter'. Into the latter category fall Alexander Garden and Miss Colden of New York, and Dr. Lining of Charleston. From Dr. Garden (and, apparently, Miss Colden) Whytt received a specimen of a plant known as *Gardenia Coldenia* in consequence of its discoverers. Whytt published an account of it, together with a description of the 'matrix or ovary of the Buccinium Ampullatum' from the same source. Dr. Lining sent an account of a yellow fever epidemic and of the vermifuge virtues of the Indian or Carolina Pink. Some account of these and of Whytt's smaller papers is given in chapter five.

Among Whytt's friends and correspondents were Stephen Hales and Sir John Pringle. He was the first to publish Hales' experiment with the decapitated frog, which was fundamental for the discovery of the reflex, and in many places he owns his debt to Hales' researches. Pringle figured in Whytt's election to the Royal Society (on 16 April 1752[32]) and persuaded him to contribute to the *Philosophical Transactions*. After Whytt's death, he helped to produce the *Works*, which Robert Whytt the younger dedicated to him 'in Testimony of the sincere Friendship that subsisted between him and the author; and in Gratitude for the Care he has taken of this complete Edition of his Works'. Perhaps Pringle had become acquainted with Whytt when they had both practised in Edinburgh. Having married the daughter of Dr. Oliver (of biscuit fame) of Bath, Pringle settled in London in 1749 and was able to keep Whytt informed when Horace Walpole began taking Whytt's medicine for the stone.

Walpole died in 1757. He, like his brother Sir Robert, had long been prey to a stone of the bladder, and though he thought himself cured, as the *Dictionary of National Biography*[33] says, 'by a remedy he sent to the Royal Society' (that is, Whytt's lime-water) 'a return of the disease early in 1757 proved fatal'. This contrasts with Pringle's letter to Whytt, in which Pringle does not seem to attribute Walpole's death to the stone: there were, when the bladder was opened, three small smooth stones, which would not be considered dangerous. Walpole, during the time he was taking Whytt's medicine, showed evidence of a diminution of his stones.

[32] I am indebted for this fact to the Librarian of the Royal Society.
[33] London, 1899, vol. 59, p. 169.

It was probably this which prompted Pringle to ask Whytt for a paper on the subject of the treatment of the stone, to be read to the Royal Society.

In 1756 Plummer retired from his post of teaching Chemistry at Edinburgh, and Whytt, Monro *primus* and Cullen combined to fulfil the duties of the post. Apart from his academic successes, says the Harveian Oration, ' . . . his success in healing disease could not fail to establish his reputation both at home and abroad'. It is certain that another of his testimonials, which was written in this year, would have lent a great deal of support to the candidate of the St. Andrews M.D. degree.

In 1761 Whytt was appointed First Physician to the King in Scotland, a post said to have been created specially for him. His antagonist in several physiological disputes, the eminent Haller, was Physician to the King, presumably while he remained south of the border. Their disagreements, which continued over several years, are dealt with in chapter six. Whytt would have been glad to hear the later enthusiastic if unqualified opinions of a member of his family: 'Dr. Whytte had a great correspondence or controversy with the celebrated German Physician Baron Haller on anatomical subjects, and he beat the baron hollow',[34] and of an Edinburgh student who scribbled in the University Library copy of the *Works*: 'I think the Doctor has fought a very good Battle, and seems to come off Conqueror'.[35] Another student, finding the same asperity in Whytt's spirited arguments that Haller had complained of, observed of the debate on sensibility and irritability that it appeared to *him* that 'neither Baron Haller nor Dr. Whytt were deficient in irritability'.[36]

At the age of forty-nine, Whytt was elected President of the Royal College of Physicians, Edinburgh. The date of his election was 1 December 1763,[37] although Bower and Dezeimeris give the year as 1764, as does the Harveian Oration. In 1764 was published Whytt's *Observations on the Nature, Causes and Cure of those Diseases which are commonly called Nervous, Hypochondriac or Hysteric: to which are prefixed Some Remarks on the Sympathy of the Nerves*. The *Dictionary of National Biography*[38] describes this as his greatest book, but it is

[34] In a letter written by Miss Betty Hamilton. Quoted by B. Balfour-Melville op. cit., p. 257.
[35] Perhaps written in 1794. It is on p. 273 of a copy of the *Works* in Edinburgh University Library, press mark G.I.12.
[36] Ibid., p. 280.
[37] I am indebted for this information to G. R. Pendrill Esq., Librarian of the Royal College of Physicians, Edinburgh.
[38] *The Dictionary of National Biography*, London, 1909, vol. 21, p. 174.

certainly of less significance than his essay on vital motions. It was well received, went through two more editions (all in Edinburgh) in 1765 and 1767, and was translated into French by Achille Guillaume Le Begue de Presle in 1767 in two volumes, and by Didot, Paris, 1777. The former included anatomical explanations of the nerves by Monro, and a bibliography of similar books. Le Begue de Presle commented upon the treatment: 'No one [but Whytt] has described the symptoms with greater accuracy, or diagnosed with greater wisdom . . . the favourable reception of the work proves that Monsieur Whytt has discovered the best methods of treatment'.[39] He stressed the importance of the book to all women, and to men of sedentary occupations. He also recommended Whytt's opinion of the nervous spirits. From an entry in Ersch's *Literatur der Medicin*, (1822)[39a] it seems that a German translation was published in Leipzig in 1766. 'Rb. WHYTT'S Beobb. üb. d. Krankhh. d. man gewölnl. Nerven—übel, ing, hypochond. u. hyster. Zufälle nennt; nach d. 2n engl. A. übers. *Lpz.*, Fritsch (766) 794 qr. 8 (1 Thl.).' With the publication of this book in 1764, Whytt's career virtually ended. His wife died in the same year, on 25 May, and in 1765 Whytt's own health began to fail. It is probable that the misfortunes of his domestic life hastened his illness; 'le chagrin qu'il en éprouva contribua sans doute à hâter son fin'.[40]

His first symptom was considerable diuresis which gradually lessened. The pulse became irregular and he was subject to attacks of depression which increased as the disease progressed; he remained indoors, driving out only on fine days. It became evident that there was a source of irritation in the alimentary canal: flatulent symptoms often gave rise to spasms of the bowels. Through the duration of the disease he coughed, producing a thick phlegm.

From an early age Whytt had had difficulty in lying on the right side,[41] and just before his illness, some gouty symptoms of a slight nature

[39] R. Whytt, *Les vapeurs et maladies nerveuses, hypochondriaques ou hystériques, reconnus et traitées dans les deux sexes*, trans. by Achille Guillame Le Begue de Presle, Paris, 1767, preface, p. v.

[39a] No. 4347. Rb. Whytt's Beobb. üb. d. Krankhh. d. man gewöhnl, Nervenübel, ingl. hypochond. u. hyster. Zwfälle nennt; nach d. Zu engl. A. über. *Lpz.*, Fritsch (766) 794 gr. 8 (1Thl.).

[40] *Biographie Universelle*, Paris, 1843, vol. 44, p. 555.

[41] On page 625 of the *Works*, Whytt describes how he was wont to suffer nightmares on account of his disordered stomach, which became worse if he lay on his back. On page 635 he remarks that he had been troubled for many years (this was published in 1764) with wind in the stomach, giddiness and faintness; he was easily startled. In his paper on the anomalous gout of 1754, he ascribed his frequent flatulence and 'faintness at the stomach' to gout. For this he prescribed, for himself and others, what was sometimes known as 'Whytt's tincture'; it is described later.

had appeared, both of which appearances lessened the apprehension of his medical advisers as to the serious nature of his afflictions; later in his illness, the difficulty of lying passed into orthopnoea. He thought himself that all his symptoms were gouty, as did Rutherford and Dr. John Clerk. Porterfield was of the opinion that they were 'hypochondriac'. Haller recorded a similar opinion in his *Bibliotheca Anatomica*.

His sense of sinking induced him to take more animal food and wine than his doctors thought wise; in the summer of that year, he developed a purple discolouration of the thighs and lower legs, as of scurvy, but without deterioration of the gums. He was put on a vegetable diet and the spots disappeared.

Two or three days before his death, perceiving that the renewed deterioration of his lower limbs was now irreversible, he said calmly to those about him, 'The end is come at last', and on 15 April 1766, in a fit of coughing, he died.

The chest and abdomen were examined after his death; in the cavity of the left pleura, there were some five pounds of fluid, mixed with a substance of gelatinous consistency and bluish colour. In the right cavity there were two pounds of serum, and on the left side, some adhesions. The lungs were free of disease, but the heart seemed atrophied and there was fluid in the pericardium. The viscera were healthy apart from a red spot the size of a shilling on the mucous membrane of the stomach. There was very little water in the abdomen, and concretions in the pancreas.

The registers of Greyfriars Church record Whytt's 'decay', and the Harveian Oration speaks of 'a tedious complication of the chronic ailments which chiefly appeared under the form of diabetes . . . '. Seller did not voice an opinion when he wrote his biographical sketch in 1862, and Barclay in 1922 said that the symptoms correspond to no known disease. Comrie[42] agreed with the Harveian Oration.

He was given a public funeral—the principal Professors of the University, in their gowns, preceded by the Mace, and the whole body of the College of Physicians—and was buried in old Greyfriars South Churchyard on the West side. The inscription on his tomb reads: Hic jacet Robertus Whytt de Bennochy, armiger, medicus regius, Med: in Acad: Edin: P., Colleg: Med: Reg: Praeses, et S.R.: S. ob. XV. Ap. MDCCLXVI. Necnon Louisa Balfour, ejus uxor quatuor decim liberorum mater ob. XXV maii M.DCCLXIV aetat. XLVI. Optimus parentibus, patri vere illustri tam humanitate

[42] J. D. Comrie, 'An eighteenth century neurologist', *Edinb. med. J.*, 1925, *32*, 755.

quam ingenio praeclaro, matri dilectissimae virtutibus quae sexum suum ornant locupleti, hocce marmor sacrum voluit Robertus Whytt de Bennochy, Armiger.[43]

The Harveian Oration says of him:

. . . he was neither an abstruse student who converted his chamber into a cloister, nor did he seek for amusement in those scenes of dissipation which are equally destructive to health . . . . He was above the middle stature, of stout and well formed make, and of a comely countenance; his manners were easy and engaging, his temper cheerful and his disposition amiable. He displayed a striking example that life is short only to the indigent insofar as it can be computed not by days or years, but by meritorious transactions. During the course of an active life not only in the uses of his profession, in relaxation from business or from study, and in private or domestic life, but in many important transactions both in the church and in the state, he demonstrated a conduct regulated by the most determined steadiness of mind, the greatest probity and the strictest honour. He was a fond father, an affectionate husband and a firm friend. He showed a steady attachment to his King and his Country, and art and zeal for the support of both civil and religious liberty. In the line of physician he was a determined practitioner, an able teacher and a judicious writer. In the line of private citizen he was an accomplished, an active, and an honest man.

Haller in his *Bibliotheca Anatomica*, observed, in the entry under 'Robertus Whytt, Professor et Medicus primarius Edinburgensis':

Since he has engaged from time to time in disputes with me, care should be taken lest my judgement of the man be affected by personal feelings. He was certainly a man of great ingenuity and perspicacity, and since he almost approached the Stahlian position of deriving all animal motions from the soul, he found myself and the mechanists opposed to him, whose opinion he considered to be necessarily unsound.

It is fairly certain that Whytt's reputation was greater on the Continent than at home, and some have been of the opinion that Whytt has suffered from an undeserved obscurity. This has been attributed to jealousy of Whytt by a colleague; Cullen's name has been mentioned. Cullen, however, deals fairly with Whytt in his works and can hardly be accused of this. Miss Betty Hamilton in a letter to James Balfour, observed of her relation:

Dr. Whytte of Bennochy, in Fife, a very eminent physician in his day, whose fame was much higher on the Continent and in

[43] J. Brown, *The Epitaphs and Monumental Inscriptions in Greyfriars Churchyard*, Edinburgh, 1867, p. 220.

London than in his native city, owing to the rivalry of the disposition of one of his contemporaries, whom I do not choose to name, who did much to cross him in his life time and suppress his fame after his death . . .[44]

Rutherford retired at about the time of the death of Whytt. His successor was Gregory instead of Cullen, who was generally expected to fill Rutherford's place. Cullen was at first unwilling to stand for election, but later accepted Whytt's chair of the theory of Medicine. Seller hints at intrigues.

Of Whytt's fourteen children by his second wife, Louisa, four died at the age of about one year, and four at the age of five years. The remaining six children survived their parents: Jean married her cousin John Balfour of Pilrig, and Martha married Major James Wilson of the Royal Artillery.

The eldest son, Robert, who like his grandfather belonged to the Faculty of Advocates of Scotland, edited and published his father's collected works in 1768, with the help of Sir John Pringle. Their policy was to render the writings less controversial, which they pursued by softening Whytt's asperity or omitting names. The book was first offered for sale on 4 January, 'Price neatly bound, one guinea'. This book, *The Works of Robert Whytt*, Edinburgh, 1768, will in the present study be referred to as the *Works*. (Whytt's *Observations on the Most Frequent Species of the Hydrocephalus Internus* was also published at the same time.) Robert died aged 27 and without family at Naples, on 22 March 1776, and the second son John succeeded.

John, who spelt his name Whyte, adopted the name Whyte-Melville on becoming heir to the entailed estates of General Melville of Strathkinness. This was the culmination of the growing relationship between the two families. Robert the physician, as shown above, was commissioned to look after the business of Lt. Melville, and two letters of John Whyte to General Melville in 1795 show that the same relationship existed with his son. John may have had legal training (although there is a John Whytt listed among the members of the Medical Society in Edinburgh, with the date 21 January 1775, there is no way of identifying him), for in 1794 and 1795 he wrote to Lord Balgonie and General

---

[44] Also: 'A late eminent physician in Edinburgh, when a young man, was employed by Dr. Whytte to assist him with some of his anatomical experiments, merely as an operative. He afterwards taught (as I was told by a physician who was no relation) the doctor's discoveries as his own. The same liberty was taken with some of his papers by a physician in Glasgow who had got hold of some of them by the imprudence of one who had access to them.' (B. Balfour-Melville, op. cit., appendix.)

15

Melville advising on technicalities in the laws of succession.[45] In 1778 or before, John Whyte in the company of General Melville and Lord Monboddo visited a Roman camp, called Re Dykes, on the Grampian Hills, near Stonehaven. Robert Barclay, the owner of the land, sent a plan of it to General Melville, and it was published posthumously, in a work by his friend, Major General Ray. There are three other maps of 1754 and one of 1778, but it is not clear whether John Whyte was similarly associated with General Melville in more examinations of the country's antiquities.

The letter of 1795 was presumably part of the arrangements concerning John Whyte as General Melville's heir, for John Whyte took the name Melville in a licence dated 24 July 1798: General Melville died in 1809, and thus John Whyte changed his name before inheriting the estates of General Melville, a point missed in biographical accounts. The Armorial Bearings were recorded in the Lyon Office on 10 May 1799.[46] This date is also wrongly given in most accounts.

He married Elizabeth, daughter of Archibald McGilchrist of North Bar in the County of Renfrew, and their son John married Lady Catherine Osborne, daughter of Francis Godolphin, the fifth Duke of Leeds. George Whyte-Melville, their son, was a popular nineteenth-century novelist whose stories of hunting and sporting life are comparable to those of Surtees. When he died in a hunting accident, the Whyte family came to an end.[47] The record of early deaths shows that the family was not characterized by robust constitution. This is perhaps unconsciously symbolized by the seal used by John Whyte-Melville on his personal correspondence: the figure of Fate removing the blossom of a flower in full bloom.

[45] There was also a letter advising General Melville about his financial affairs. Copies exist in the Scottish Record Office.
[46] A copy of a licence affirming this record is among the papers of E. W. M. Balfour-Melville, in the Scottish Record Office.
[47] There were of course many female lines. George Whyte-Melville himself married the Hon. Charlotte Hanbury (daughter of the first Lord Bateman) and was the father of four daughters. There remained however no one to call Bennochy the family seat in the male line, and the house had been pulled down as early as 1835.

16

CHAPTER II

The Controversy with Alston:
Black and Whytt

Events of the 1740s reveal the widespread occurrence of and consequent interest in the stone of the bladder. The sufferer was faced with the choice between attempting to ameliorate this painful condition with repugnant medicines of doubtful efficacy for perhaps the rest of his life and the horrors of a lithotomy. Any effective treatment would solve this painful dilemma, and when Mrs. Stephens cured the Postmaster General, it seemed to many that salvation was at hand.[1] The conditions attached to her Parliamentary grant were that the medicine was to be investigated by a panel of eminent trustees, including David Hartley, William Cheselden and Stephen Hales. They met in March, 1740, with the exception of Sir Robert Walpole (had he attended he might have preferred this medicine to Jurin's dangerous lixivium which probably killed him) and interviewed cured sufferers and their physicians. Hales had already tried to find a solvent for the stone, and now, with Hartley, he experimented with this medicine to attempt to separate the active constituents from the burnt wild carrot and burdock seeds and other irrelevancies. They both published their results,[2] which were read by Whytt, Alston and Rutty, who like their authors, fastened on the lime-water as the 'grand essential Article',[3] aided by soap. Jurin's ill-fated suggestion that soap lye—the very caustic alkaline constituent of soap—could be taken internally rather than indirectly in soap and lime-water, was published with Rutty's tract.

As a former pupil of Cheselden, now a trustee, Whytt was doubtless eager to find an alternative to lithotomy. Deciding that the lime-water was more important than the soap, he seized the first

[1] See A. E. Clark-Kennedy, *Stephen Hales, D.D., F.R.S. An Eighteenth Century Biography*, Cambridge, 1929, pp. 124–30. See also pp. 5, 6 above.

[2] Details are given in Henry Guerlac, 'Joseph Black and Fixed Air. A bicentenary retrospective, with some new or little known material', *Isis*, 1957, **48**, 139. Black was also influenced by Hales, Ibid., p. 148.

[3] J. Rutty, *An Account of some new Experiments and Observations on Joanna Stephens's Medicine for the Stone: to which is subjoined An Account of the Effects of Soap-Lees taken internally, in the Case of James Jurin, M.D.*, London, 1742, p. ii.

17

opportunity of putting it to the test, which occurred in the person of David Millar, very probably Whytt's old schoolmaster. Medicines since 1704 had been unavailing until Whytt prescribed lime-water in 1741: its success encouraged him to publish his *Essay* in 1744, probably read to the Medical Society in 1743 (see above, p. 6). Rescuing Mrs. Stephen's potion from 'the Imputation of being merely Empirical'[4] was clearly thought important, and the *Essay* helped Whytt to his chair at Edinburgh, where Alston had been making lime-water since 1743 for horticulture.

He begins by reviewing the work of Hales, Hartley, Rutty and Jurin. Like Hales he thought the soap useful only because it contained lime, and having discovered that Alicant soap was made without lime, he was led to the lime-water. He mixed quick-lime with various liquids to determine that water was in fact the best vehicle for its virtues; he added lime-water to urine to show that it prevented the latter forming crusts; and he demonstrated the 'dissolving' power of lime-water on a stone in an open vessel. A possible explanation of the controversy with Alston over the 'strength' of lime-water is that Alston's was more concentrated— probably saturated—than Whytt's early lime-water. Calcium hydroxide is less soluble in hot than cold water and Whytt, slaking the lime with eight or ten times its weight of boiling water[5] and hardly allowing time for cooling (four or five hours in this first edition, three or four in the 1747 edition[6]), doubtless produced weaker lime-water than that of Alston's cold water slaking. When Whytt used the latter method the lime-water was 'more harsh and disagreeable'[7] so perhaps it was more concentrated. Moreover he usually conducted his experiments on its action on the stone at a moderate heat[8], unlike Alston.[9]

Their differences in chemistry were more important. Hales had suggested that the 'sulphureous and elastick' particles of fire are fixed in lime during calcination and are released on slaking, generating heat. They were analogous to the fixed air, which, becoming elastic, was driven off from oyster shells and chalk in

[4] Ibid., p. iii.
[5] 1744 ed., p. 683. The various editions of the paper will be referred to by their dates.
[6] 1744 ed., p. 693, and the second ed., *Medical Essays and Observations*, 1747, 5, part 2, 130.
[7] 1744 ed., p. 693.
[8] This was between body temperature and the melting point of wax, perhaps 100°F. (1744 ed., pp. 692, 736.) Perhaps, like Black, he wanted a heat 'pretty near the animal'. (Guerlac, op. cit., p. 148.)
[9] C. Alston, *A Dissertation on Quick Lime and Lime Water*, Edinburgh, 1752, p. 35.

calcination.[10] Whytt thought the 'fiery Particles'[11] of quick-lime could be 'sheathed' by oil, but that they remained active in the water used in slaking and were liable to escape when the lime-water was exposed to air, allowing the earthy particles of lime to come together and form a crust. In later editions he attributes lithontripticity to the fire particles of lime-water but here he assigns it to the *lime* particles, held in solution by fire particles.[12] Particles of lime in oyster-shell lime-water, he argues from experiments, are more powerful than those of stone lime.[13] Further experiments show that lime-water is unaffected by the animal humours—its properties remain intact on its way to the bladder—but vitiated by certain medicines, drinks, and foods. Three pints of it should be drunk every day.

In the 1747 edition he observes that the water with which he slaked the calcined shells was specifically heavier afterwards.[14] Langrish had boiled lime-water to dryness and found less calcarious matter than Whytt expected from its specific gravity, and Whytt concluded that some 'very active volatile Matter', i.e., fire particles, had evaporated with the water. Examining the crust formed on exposed lime-water, he considered it a quite insipid *'alcali terreux'*[15] so he now thought the *fire* particles of lime-water were lithontriptic.

The enlarged paper was published separately in Edinburgh in 1752 as *An Essay on the Virtues of Lime-Water in the Cure of the Stone.* Hales had written to Whytt suggesting that lime-water would be more lithontriptic if poured again on freshly-calcined oyster shells. Whytt made a series of 'double' lime-waters thus and found their specific gravities correspondingly greater than 'single'. He now took a day or two in making single lime-water, depending on the proportion of water to shell-lime, which contrasts with the earlier three or four hours and suggests the solution was nearing saturation, particularly as he finds he can make effective lime-water when the proportion of water to lime is as great as 270 to 1.

A few months later came Alston's first *Dissertation.* Alston had previously found that a pound of quick-lime yielded 400 lbs. of lime-water, and now shows the ratio can be extended to 1 to 590, the last of a series of infusions being as strong as the first. He argues

[10] S. Hales, *Vegetable Staticks*, London, 1727 (reprinted 1961 by Oldbourne), pp. 96, 98, 101, 162.

[11] 1744 ed., p. 682. Rutty, op. cit., pp. 11, 12 also accepts the fire particle theory.

[12] But the fire particles of a quick-lime potash mixture are lithontriptic. 1744 ed., pp. 717, 710.

[13] Ibid., p. 722. Its particles are more 'subtile saponaceous and penetrating'.

[14] 1747 ed., p. 197. It was heavier than water by 1/212, a large difference, later reduced.

[15] Ibid., pp. 197, 198, 201.

that lime has an upper limit to its solubility, so 'double' could not be stronger than 'single' lime-water, as both were saturated, or should be: he later observed of Whytt 'There are other Circumstances as necessary to the compleat Saturation of the Water, which seem to have been neglected'.[16] He had told Whytt of his discovery that a pound of lime would yield several hundred pounds of lime-water, each equally strong, and was annoyed not to find himself mentioned in the 1752 edition of the *Essay* where Whytt uses water 270 times the weight of the lime: 'So I claim the discovery; though Dr. Whytt has not done me the Honour to mention me for it'.[17]

Alston measured the strength of lime-water by allowing it to form a crust in the air. When no more formed after stirring, and the liquid no longer turned syrup of violets green, vegetable infusions yellow, or corrosive sublimate red (Whytt thought claret would detect lime after these tests failed), he weighed the crust, which he found the same for any similar volume of any lime-water, and more than the lime in solution: he concluded that half its weight came from the terrestrial parts of the water, or from the air, thus almost anticipating Black's discovery.[18] He could find no difference between the specific gravities of lime-water and common water before slaking.

Whytt replied in the *Essays and Observations, Physical and Literary*, (1754), **1**, 372, with more experiments undertaken with the help of James Gray, 'Of the various Strength of different Lime waters'. These experiments were principally concerned with specific gravity measurements, although Alston had already pointed out[19] the difficulty of obtaining accurate results, and that the most that could be expected was a difference of one part in a thousand between the weight of a volume of lime-water and of the same volume of pure water. An alternative method was to weigh a glass globe in the liquids—Black seems to have preferred this method[20]—and Whytt and Alston argued bitterly about the imperfections of the other's apparatus.

Whytt and Gray's results were confirmed by titrations of the waters against claret (which was neutralized when it turned the colour of gun-powder) and by weighing the precipitate obtained by adding salt of tartar to lime-water. Alston observed that the

---

[16] C. Alston, *A Second Dissertation on Quick Lime and Lime Water*, Edinburgh, 1755, p. 27.

[17] First *Dissertation*, p. 47. See also pp. 4, 53. Alston had also communicated his discovery to the Royal Society. Guerlac, op. cit., p. 145.

[18] Ibid., pp. 8, 9. See also Guerlac, op. cit., pp. 138, 146.

[19] First *Dissertation*, p. 48.   [20] Guerlac, op. cit., pp. 149, 150.

wine varied too much from year to year to be dependable, and that the latter precipitate was entirely from the tartar, the strength of which alone it measured. Whytt's argument was an 'Attempt to prove, that we see not what we see'.[21]

After Whytt and Gray came Black, who in that year published his doctoral thesis at Edinburgh. Black had arrived from Glasgow (and Cullen) in 1752 already interested in lime-water, in the possibility of dissolving the stone and in the fire particle theory.[22] Cullen, who knew Alston's work, had suggested to Black the chemistry of lime and lime-water as a thesis topic. Once in Edinburgh, Black changed his mind, to avoid entering Whytt and Alston's dispute and appearing 'presumptuous'.[23] He retained his medical purpose in trying to find a solvent for the stone stronger than lime-water and cast around for a suitable chemical substance. Whytt's ideas had first put the notion into his mind: 'Dr. Whytt imagined that he had discovered that the lime-water of oyster-shell lime had more power as a solvent, than the lime-water of common stone lime. I therefore conceived hopes that, by trying a greater variety of the alkaline earths, some kinds might be found still more different by their qualities from the common kind; and perhaps yielding a lime-water still more powerful than that of oyster-shell lime'.[24]

Even before this, it was probably Whytt's *Essay* that prompted Black to make some experiments to test the theory of fire particle causticity, which he abandoned as a result. In his lectures he is recorded as saying 'The disputes that arrose betwixt Dr. Whytt and Alston of the best lime for making lime-water engaged me to make some Expts. if I could find out a Lime from some Absorbt. Earth & the 1st that offered itself was the *Magnes: Alb:*'[25] His thesis (quoting approvingly the 'celebrated professors Whytt and Alston'[26]) suggests that fixed air is driven from magnesia alba in calcination and can be replaced by the reaction of a salt of the magnesia with an alkali. The cycle of reactions began again with the recalcination of the precipitate. The salt could also be produced by driving the air from the magnesia alba with an acid. As the calcined magnesia alba did not slake like quick-lime nor produce a lime-water, Black

[21] First *Dissertation*, 2nd ed., Edinburgh, 1754, p. 64.
[22] Guerlac, op. cit., pp. 134, 148. Black wrote to Cullen saying he had been too busy to read 'one word on Lime-water', as he had intended.
[23] Ibid., pp. 149, 150.
[24] Ibid., p. 151.
[25] T. Cochrane, *Notes from Doctor Black's lectures on Chemistry 1767/8*, ed. D. McKie, Wilmslow, I.C.I. Ltd., 1968, p. 65.
[26] J. Black, *Dissertatio Medica Inauguralis de Humore Acido a Cibis Orto, et Magnesia Alba*, Edinburgh, 1754, p. 288. (In W. Smellie, ed., *Thesaurus Medicus*, Edinburgh, 1779.)

was 'disappointed in my expectations'[27] and his original purpose had to be abandoned.

In the second edition of his *Dissertation*, later that year, Alston uses Black's figures on the quantity of magnesia that destroys the properties of a volume of lime-water to defend his statement that the crust formed on lime-water is greater than the lime dissolved. He brings forward new arguments against Whytt's notions of double lime-water, which reveal a weakness in Whytt's method of making it. Whytt had measured its strength by its lithontripticity and specific gravity. Alston[28] undertakes to show that the high specific gravity is due to impurities from imperfectly calcined shells. His own 'quadruple' lime-water was heavier than single by reason of soluble impurities discoverable by determining the specific gravity before and after the crust had formed, the latter being the same in weight as in single lime-water. Whytt often found sea salt still in the shells after calcination[29], and the sulphureous smell during calcination, which he first thought came from the coal and only later from the shells themselves,[30] imparted to the lime-water a disagreeable taste and an ability to turn silver a copper colour. No doubt this remaining organic matter and salt confused Whytt's results. Guerlac seems to suggest he falsified some of them.[31]

In the second edition of the separate *Essay*, 1755, Whytt says there is 'inconsiderable' difference between lime-waters made with water twelve, and eight times the weight of lime *provided* sufficient time is allowed; it was neglecting this that led to his earlier error. Here he has clearly been influenced by Alston's many successive infusions: he justifies his earlier silence on Alston's discovery by saying it was 'partly real and partly imaginary',[32] still insisting that each successive infusion up to his own total of 270:1 and Alston's 500:1 in water to lime, is slightly weaker.[33] (Nevertheless, his lime

[27] J. Black, 'Experiments upon Magnesia alba, Quicklime, and some other Alcaline Substances', *Essays and Observations, Physical and Literary*, 1756, 2, 160.

[28] First *Dissertation*, 2nd ed., p. 59. His quadruple lime-water was that which had slaked four separate quantities of quick-lime.

[29] 1744 ed., pp. 711, 721, 1755 ed., pp. 52, 83.

[30] 1747 ed., p. 180. 1752 ed., p. 34.

[31] Guerlac, op. cit., p. 144. That the impurities were more soluble than lime might explain the specific gravity decrease in successive infusions. Whytt weighed a glass phial in the liquids, helped by John Stuart, the professor of natural philosophy at Edinburgh. His strongest, 'double' lime-water was as to pure water 169:168. Lime that had already given 100 times its weight of lime-water (double lime-water being made from fresh quick-lime) was 926: 925 a better figure. (See Guerlac, op. cit., p. 144.)

[32] 1775 ed., pp. 34, 44.

[33] Contamination by carbon dioxide might account for this. The falling off in strength was less in lime-water in closed vessels. 1755 ed., pp. 48–50.

water must now have been saturated.[34]) He was now firmly opposed to Black and Alston on the concept of maximum solubility of lime and less firmly on the fire particle theory, to which indeed, he had never been wholly committed.[35]

The next publication was Alston's *Second Dissertation* in the same year, 1755. After noting with approval Black's experiments on lime, 'which seem to throw more light on that obscure substance, than all the labours of the Chymists have done hitherto' and with disapproval Whytt's criticism of his own experiments—'he has animadverted pretty smartly upon some of them'[36]—he devotes the entire book to an attack on Whytt's ideas on single, double, stone and shell lime-waters, the reaction with salt of tartar and the fire particle theory. The arguments are developed from the first *Dissertation*, reinforced by more experiments and a quantitative approach which compares well with Whytt's.

It is probable that this approach owes something to Black. The mutual influence of Black and Alston is noted by Guerlac, who has however, missed an important point. Although Black thought Alston not 'a good enough chemist to be perfect in his profession',[37] he followed him in the preparation of quick-lime, in testing for lime-water and in not using heat for the magnesia-lime water reaction. It has already been noted how it was Whytt's work that first determined the course of Black's investigations, and we must assume there was some communication between all three during this period. Black wrote to Cullen after his thesis was published observing that Alston was pleased with it, and Alston's dissertation contains several approving references to it: in refuting Whytt that quick-lime and soap-lye are very corrosive because of a transfer of fire particles from the lime to the lye, Alston observes of Black, 'This gentleman's Experiments which we hope to see soon made public, will no doubt explain this, and several other things concerning the nature of quick-lime, which were perhaps never thought of before';[38] he asked Black, who happened to call in, to estimate the strength of lime-water by taste;[39] his salt of tartar

[34] Modern calculations (assuming pure reagents) suggest that the precipitate from salt of tartar and lime-water is approximately correct for a saturated solution. 1755 ed., p. 46.

[35] His caution is seen in the 1747 ed., p. 201, 1752 ed., p. 77, and 1755 ed., pp. 95 and 77 where he argues from Black's thesis that exposed lime-water grows weaker not by losing fire particles but by absorbing air.

[36] *Second Dissertation*, pp. v, vi.   [37] Guerlac, op. cit., p. 441.

[38] *Second Dissertation*, p. 53. He also speaks of Black's thesis as 'an extraordinary Progress in Chymistry, and particularly his knowledge of the Quality of Lime-Water'. First *Dissertation*, 2nd ed., p. 62.

[39] First *Dissertation*, 2nd ed., p. 62.

23

was always prepared by Black;[40] and Black is in the background when Alston corrects a small mistake about magnesia alba in his second edition. Yet Alston either misunderstood the significance of Black's work on magnesia or changed his mind after Black made it clearer and extended it to lime in his 'Experiments'. While Whytt recognized the importance of fixed air in destroying the action of lime-water, Alston was concerned only with the quantitative precision of this experiment in Black's thesis, as we have seen.

Black's 'Experiments upon Magnesia Alba, Quicklime and some other Alcaline Substances' duly appeared in 1756. It was a general statement on the chemistry of alkalis[41] derived from his thesis and extended particularly to lime. The causticity of quick-lime was due to its lack of fixed air; it had no fire particles and was a uniform earthy substance which should therefore be totally soluble in water, with a maximum solubility. He had thought total solubility would be difficult to prove. Some encouragement was available from Alston's[42] novel long series of lime-waters, but none from Whytt's work. Black omits the reference to Whytt and Alston here, and in later lectures he attributed to Alston as well as Whytt a belief in fire particle causticity,[43] so Alston's influence could not have been very profound.

Having had no reply from Whytt, Alston devoted his third *Dissertation* to an attempt to refute Black's conclusions. He and Hales had shown that there *was* lime in soap-lye, despite what Whytt had said about fixed fire and Black about fixed air. Quick-lime was not caustic through lack of fixed air, nor did it make soap-lye caustic by attracting its fixed air: 'Whatever attraction Therefore Quick-Lime may have for fixed air, it is not by it soon reduced to an inactive calcarious earth'.[44] No, quick-lime makes alkaline salts and lye caustic by removing from them part of their earth, 'to say nothing' of what it gives them of its own principles. Nor was fixed air limited to alkalis, and in a mixture of acids and alkalis the escaping air could equally come from the acids, for despite Black, air and acid could be 'conjoined to the same body'.[45] Alston confuses the effervescence of escaping 'air' with the

[40] *Second Dissertation*, p. 46.
[41] Guerlac, op. cit., has a full account of Black's work, for which there is not room here.
[42] Alston had said only a third part of lime was soluble. First *Dissertation*, p. 11.
[43] Guerlac, op. cit., p. 442.
[44] C. Alston, *A Third Dissertation on Quick-Lime and Lime Water*, Edinburgh, 1757, p. 9. Guerlac misses this and Whytt's 1761 ed. (also in the *Works*) and represents Whytt as opposed to Black and Alston, while in fact Whytt agreed with Black and both disagreed with Alston over the role of fixed air.
[45] Ibid., p. 14.

24

ebullition of strong reagents, and misses the importance of the role of fixed air—he refers to 'that curious Experiment whereby the Doctor produced . . . Quick-lime without fire'[46]—and thought that Black's results were due to persistent impurities. His taste for debate emerges in his attacks on the 'Edinburgh Reviewer', the *Critical Review* and papers by Schlosser and Springfield,[47] who thought the Carlsbad waters six times as lithontriptic as lime-water. Springfield specifically rejected Whytt's views, who published some rather inconclusive experiments in reply the next year.[48]

Whytt had the last word with the third edition of his separate *Essay* in 1761. Recognizing Black's abilities as a chemist, whose account of the chemistry of quick-lime and lime-water was 'equally new and satisfactory',[49] Whytt abandoned the fire particle theory. He simply translated 'fire particles' into 'lack of fixed air'; quick-lime made soap-lye caustic by attracting its fixed air, rather than by fire particles moving in the opposite direction, and this causticity was not due to any lime in the lye, as Alston maintained. The fixed air theory also explained why lime lost weight in calcination[50] but emphasized the discrepancy between the specific gravity of lime-water and the weight of its dry residue. He also tailors the theory to account for the lithontripticity of lime-water: it attracts fixed air from the stone (and not oil, as he thought earlier). He no longer thinks shell-lime particles are more saponaceous and subtle, and he abandons claret titrations, both as a result of Alston's criticism.

A minor topic on which Alston and Whytt agreed was that lime-water would not dissolve all stones. They both found in their experiments that certain rare, dark-coloured and hard stones were quite uninfluenced by lime-water.[51] Hales had already noticed them,[52] and they were probably the same as the mulberry-stones of Morand and Rutty.[53] Dr. Lobb found that lime-water would dissolve no stones at all, which Whytt explained by the experiments being made in winter, taking care that his own were performed in warmer weather.[54]

As well as pursuing the oral administration of lime-water, Whytt was interested in more direct methods. He knew that Hales and Le Dran had introduced liquid into the bladders of a bitch and a

[46] Ibid., p. 11.
[47] Springfield's paper is to be found in *Phil.Trans.*, 1755–6, **49**, 895.
[48] *Phil.Trans.*, 1757–8, **50**, 386.
[49] *Works*, p. 385.
[50] Alston had argued that the added fire particles would have to have had negative weight. *Second Dissertation*, p. 54.
[51] Alston, *First Dissertation*, p. 38. Whytt, *Works*, p. 422.
[52] Guerlac, op. cit., p. 140.
[53] Rutty, op. cit., p. vii.   [54] *Works*, p. 351.

human patient respectively,[55] and no doubt from his student days with Cheselden he knew that warm water was often injected 'in order to the high Operation for the Stone'[56] and he suggested that lime-water could also be injected. A catheter was the usual instrument for these operations, and Whytt suggested that a flexible catheter could be retained in the bladder to avoid the pain caused by a frequent insertion.

Langrish read the first edition of Whytt's essay, and took up the suggestion, successfully injecting lime-water into the bladder of a dog twice a day for a month. In the second edition, Whytt describes[57] how he requested the surgeon Campbell to perform the same operation upon a boy awaiting a lithotomy, which he did, in 1745. Whytt found the catheter unsuitable, notwithstanding its flexibility, and suggested that an ivory pipe 'with a Sheeps-bladder tied upon its great End'[58] might be used to greater advantage. Advice from friends made him defer an experiment with such a device until 1752, when he asked a medical student, Butter, to help him. Together they evolved a mechanism involving a tin tube and an ox bladder charged with lime-water, and a satisfactory technique.[59] An alternative was to employ 'Mr. Daran's newly invented hollow *bougie*'.[60]

[55] 1744 ed., p. 734.
[56] Ibid.
[57] 1747 ed., pp. 227.

[58] Ibid., p. 228
[59] *Works*, pp. 413, 414.
[60] Ibid., p. 417

CHAPTER III

Hydrocephalus

Whytt was the first to describe accurately that species of dropsy of the brain in children, which he called hydrocephalus internus and which is now called tuberculous meningitis. His paper *Observations on the most frequent Species of the Hydrocephalous Internus, viz. the Dropsy of the Ventricles of the Brain*, was first published after his death, in Edinburgh (1768) and in the *Works*.

In common with most of his larger essays, Whytt begins with an historical introduction, which serves to show the inadequacies in the contemporary opinions which he proposes to remedy. Of the two types of dropsy, internal and external to the cranium, Whytt tells us that the former is either between the brain and the skull or within the ventricles of the brain. Hydrocephalus within the brain was the most frequent but the least well known. neither Hippocrates, Celsus, Aëtius nor Paulus Aegineta knew of it, but all admitted there was a condition of water *on* the brain. The first to conceive the possibility of true internal hydrocephalus was Hieronymous Mercuralis at the beginning of the sixteenth century. Wepfer and Boerhaave knew the condition but did not offer a list of symptoms, while Petit in 1718 furthered the matter by postmortem examinations and listing these symptoms: convulsions of mouth and eyelids, biting the lips, teeth grinding, picking the nose, looseness or costiveness of the bowels, drowsiness, dull and protruding eyes, softening of bones and opening of sutures in the skull.

Whytt observed that the list was neither complete nor diagnostic, disagreeing in particular about the swelling of the head, which, he said, could only happen in those very young children whose sutures had not yet closed. The incomplete accounts of Le Dran and Donald Monro complete Whytt's historical introduction.

Whytt's list of symptoms in the progress of the disease was taken from his case-reports of twenty children. He recognized three stages in the disease, and performed post-mortem examinations.

The first stage began with the appearance of the first recognizable symptom, four to six weeks before the termination of the disease in death. The patient was pale and emaciated, with a very high temperature and a pulse of a hundred to a hundred-and-forty.

There was a lack of appetite and spirits. Many of the symptoms of this stage resembled those of a fever caused by worms: there was aversion to light, vomiting daily or every two days and headaches (specifically, on forehead and crown; worse at night). In his essay on the sympathy of the nerves, Whytt described an itching of the nose as a sympathetic reaction to intestinal worms; here it was not described as a symptom of the fever which resembles that generated by worms, but he included it in the symptoms of the first stage of dropsy. The other symptoms were: thirst and costiveness, a grinding of the teeth and the white or clean tongue developing an aphthous redness. The patients were languid and often sleepless.

The second stage began some two to three weeks before death, and was recognized by the dropping of the pulse to about sixty (rather less than in health) and becoming irregular in both the frequency and power of its strokes. The skin nevertheless retained the same temperature, and the other symptoms of the first stage continued. The patients vomited more often and had difficulty in sitting upright; towards the end of this stage they began to grow drowsy, and their eyes developed a squint. They often moaned, but were unable to say why; fright took the place of oppression and delirium began. Worms, or something that looked like dissolved worms were voided towards the end of this stage, which occasioned them no relief, and confused their doctors into believing that these were the cause of the feverish symptoms.

Whytt seemed to distinguish between the real worms thus voided and the appearance of 'dissolved' worms, which he apparently considered to be of a different nature. It is probable that intestinal worms were more widespread in the eighteenth century than now, and any violent spasm of the bowels would have dislodged a portion of its community.

The urine in the second stage may have a white sediment, and the breath a very nauseous and offensive smell.

The secondary rise of the pulse to a feverish and regular level indicated the arrival of the third stage, about a week before death. Almost all such pulses were above a hundred and thirty, and some might reach two hundred; it gradually increased until the termination of the disease. The patients were now comatose and often suffered delusions. Paralysis of one or both eyelids was accompanied by inflammation of the conjunctiva and by a dilation of the pupils. The eyes became totally insensible a few days before death.

Respiration became difficult, with a pause after expiration. The hand was constantly raised to the head, and convulsions of the limbs became more frequent. One cheek may have been hot and the other cold. The bowels were loose.

The third stage ended in death. Whytt opened the heads of ten patients and discovered two to five ounces of water in the anterior ventricles of the brain, below the corpus callosum, and often some in the third and fourth ventricle. In no case did he meet with water between the dura mater and brain, between the hemispheres, or above the corpus callosum.

He observed that the 'water' did not coagulate with heat, like serum or lymph in the pericardium, or the fluid derived from tapping a dropsy of the abdomen.

Whytt carefully noted those diagnostic symptoms which enabled the hydrocephalus to be distinguished from a fever due to worms, or foulness of the stomach, or 'slow fever ending in a coma'. If the patient was under fifteen, with a slow irregular fever, vomiting once a day or in two days, avoiding the light, and with a continuous pain in the crown of the head, no relief being derived from purges or blisters, then such a youth could be suffering from worms or foulness of the stomach and bowels. But when the pulse dropped, and other signs of fever continued, then the illness could be identified as dropsy of the brain. This was confirmed by the appearances of heat and thirst, sleeplessness, strabismus and double vision, delirium and screaming. Identification became positive when the patient became comatose, the pupils dilated and the pulse quickened. The cheeks became flushed, and the sensitivity of the tendons gave rise finally to convulsions.

Whytt speculated about the causes of the dropsy. He concluded that the 'exhalant arteries' throw out a greater quantity of fluids than the absorbent or 'bibulous' veins can take up. He believed, as expressed elsewhere, that some of the ultimate ends of the capillaries terminated in small pores, not large enough to pass the corpuscles, while others were continuous with arterioles and small veins. In the brain, then, there may have been in such cases an original laxity of structure leading to this condition, or some injury may have been sustained during birth. Alternatively, a tumour might have compressed the absorbent veins; Petit often found a schirrhous pituitary, and Whytt found a tumour of the *thalamus nervorum opticorum*. Finally, Whytt postulated, the blood may have been too thin, and its rate of leaving the exhalant arteries greater than its absorption. Suppression of urine could have led to this condition: Whytt found that adults dying of ischuria often had water in the brain, but in relatively small quantities. Other tedious chronic diseases may have led to the condition.

The last section of the paper is headed: 'An Attempt to Account for Some of the most remarkable Symptoms attending Dropsy of the Brain'. All symptoms, he concluded, were due to pressure upon the brain by the collected water. Thus the irritated brain excites a reaction in the stomach by reason of its sympathy with that organ, in a way similar to that whereby wounds of the head often excite vomiting. The aversion to light is a result of the irritation of *thalamus nervorum opticorum* and the action of the water in the case of the heart is to slow its action by compressing its nerves: it is thus less sensible of the returning blood which normally excites it into action. On this basis, Whytt found it more difficult to explain the secondarily fast heart-beat of the third stage. He suggested that irritation of the nerves followed the weakening effect of compression. This indicates that Whytt thought of the cardiac nerves as originating in the brain, and that the stimulation of the heart by returning blood operated by way of this organ, a point he does not make equally clear in his essay on vital motions. In that essay, too, Whytt first described what has since been called 'Whytt's reflex'; that is the contraction of the pupil due to the influence of light upon the retina, acting by way of the nerves. Here Whytt shows that destruction of function of the *thalamus nervorum opticorum* by compression blocks this nervous pathway, and the pupil dilates to its position of rest. Similarly the pause in respiration after the end of expiration is due to the 'sentient principle', being less easily aroused, by reason of the pathological state of the nerves, from its 'lethargic state'. The relationship between sense, motor organs, nerves and the sentient principle is discussed later.

Whytt concluded that the disease was incurable. By its nature it could not be operated upon, and it did not show itself early enough to admit of treatment by which the more usual forms of dropsy were cured: purgatives and diuretics, frictions and blisters, exercise and dieting.

CHAPTER IV

Nervous Diseases

The book *Observations on the Nature, Causes and Cure of those Diseases which are commonly called Nervous, Hypochondriac or Hysteric; to which are prefixed some Remarks on the Sympathy of the Nerves* was published in 1764 in Edinburgh, and incorporated many of the elements of Whytt's doctrine of the behaviour of the soul, which he evolved in his essay on vital motions of animals and his controversy with Haller.

Yet apart from the prefatory chapter on the structure and sympathy of the nerves, Whytt writes primarily as a practising doctor; his interest is in the treatment of the diseases, and his efforts to understand the causes are directed toward that end. He recommends only those treatments of which he had first-hand knowledge or good authority.

The first chapter, on the structure and sympathy of the nerves, is of great interest. Whytt played a considerable part in the development of the reflex theory, as will be seen later, and what is now called reflex was for Whytt a special case of sympathy. G. S. Hall[1] thought that the doctrine of sympathy, with an immaterial communicating principle, delayed the discovery of the reflex, and it is certain that they were closely associated; Whytt put both sympathy and the other involuntary motions of animals on the same footing—nerves communicating through a central, unconscious and necessarily acting sentient principle. Most of the examples he took to illustrate sympathy were organs of the viscera— he was at particular pains to illustrate the sympathies of the uterus and intestine, whence hysteric and hypochondriac diseases, in men and women respectively, were classically supposed to originate— just as the modern sympathetic or autonomic nervous system is that which innervates the viscera, just as unconsciously and necessarily as did Whytt's soul. He thus reached a position from where the strict distinction between sympathetic actions, the reflex, and actions involuntary through habit (which he described accurately) would have been a matter of further description alone.[2]

[1] F. Fearing, *Reflex Action*, London, 1930, p. 3.
[2] In this as in other things (for example the essay on hydrocephalus), Whytt seems to stand at the threshold of the nineteenth century, and it was the

31

Sympathy, Whytt tells us, was mentioned by Hippocrates, and Galen thought it was due to the movement of humours in the body, rather than to the influence of the nerves. Fernel and Sennert followed Galen, while Du Laurens ascribed the sympathy of the uterus and mammae to the 'intercostal' nerve and azygos vein. Bauhin, Riolan and Riverius suggested that sympathy was due to continuity of veins and membranes and in addition followed a more general statement that there were five causes of sympathy: connection, situation, vicinity, similarity of parts and similarity of function.

Whytt mentions these authors principally to emphasize the novelty of his approach to sympathy. As an historical introduction it is poor: not only had Galen described many kinds of non-humoral visceral sympathy,[3] but he had attributed the chief of these to the 'sixth pair', that is, the vagus.[4] Further, he had described the sympathetic trunk in some detail.[5] Fernel[6] and Du Laurens,[7] it is true, took several examples of moving humours as causes of sympathy from Galen, but were also concerned with the structure and function of the 'intercostal' nerve. Riolan,[8] indeed, was perhaps the first to rescue this nerve from its position as a branch of the vagus, where Vesalius had put it.

The prevailing opinion at the time of Whytt was based upon that of Willis. He had described the all-important 'intercostal' nerve, distinguished from the others by its slender origins and later bulk, as a separate nervous stock.[9] By its unique combinations with the spinal nerves and manifold contributions to various nervous plexuses among the viscera, Willis held that it was the principal contributor to visceral sympathy. The intercostal was given the

descriptive science of that century which substantiated many of his ideas. Fulton observes '. . . the full implications of his doctrines did not come to be appreciated until the nineteenth century' (J. F. Fulton, 'The historical contribution of physiology to neurology', Science Medicine and History, Essays in Honour of Charles Singer, ed. E. A. Underwood, Oxford, 1963, vol. 2, p. 537).

[3] For example, Galen, De affectorum locorum notitiae, Venice, 1510, bk. 3, p. xvi.

[4] For example, Galen, De usu partium corporis humani, Paris, 1528, p. 273.

[5] Galen, On Anatomical Procedures, trans. W. Duckworth, Cambridge, 1962, p. 217. The relevant books of this work were not available to Whytt, but there were at least two current versions of The Dissection of the Nerves.

[6] J. Fernel, Universa Medicina, 4th ed., 1656, Utrecht, p. 156.

[7] A. Du Laurens, Opera Anatomica, Lyons, 1593, p. 272.

[8] J. Riolan, the younger, Anatomia (In J. Riolan, the elder, Opera Omnia, Paris, 1610, p. 112.)

[9] T. Willis, The Anatomy of the Brain, p. 157. (In the Remaining Medical Works of that Famous and Renowned Physician Dr. Thomas Willis, trans. S. Pordage, London, 1681, p. 157.)

name of 'grande sympathique' in 1732 by Winslow[10] on the same assumption, but the name was long in being accepted in Scotland; it is in fact the sympathetic trunk.

Whytt was wrong, therefore, in refusing to acknowledge the function of this nerve. During the eighteenth century, likewise following Willis, attention had centred on the plexuses and ganglia associated with the intercostal nerve, and Whytt, insisting that no kind of interaction was possible between nerves from their origin to destination, could not allow the ganglia any sympathetic function. Nevertheless, there were many of Whytt's contemporaries who believed that sympathy was due to blood vessels, continuity of membranes or the *cela cellulosa*, or even similarity of parts, and it is to his credit that he evolved a rationalized system of sympathy which, if not exclusively concerned with the viscera, was wide enough to place him in the forefront of the development of the idea of the reflex.

It is this system that we shall use to follow Whytt's paper on nervous diseases, and in a later chapter the separation of reflexes from sympathetic motions will be examined.

The central point of his doctrine was that all sympathy presupposed feeling, which could not exist without nerves. All nerves were unbranched from origin to termination, lest there be confusion of sense and motion. Their origin was the brain and spinal cord, where lay the sentient principle. *All sympathy, therefore, was effected by the intervention of the soul.*

The idea that nerve fibres are unbranched throughout their length reaches from Galen to Astruc and Albinus, Whytt's teacher, and it is worthwhile to see how Whytt uses it to refute the growing body of speculation on a system of nerves serving sympathy. There were two principal connections between nerves postulated by the rather mechanically-minded physiologists of the day (it was this mechanism to which Whytt objected): that provided by two or more nerves being involved in a common membrane at or near their origin, and that which occurred along their length in ganglia and plexuses.

Any common membrane, argued Whytt, possessing no sense and no motion, could transfer no known effect from one nerve to another. His second argument he used also against a connection by way of the ganglia: in such a simple device, there seems to be no reason why the connection should not operate in both directions. That is, two organs, sharing branches of the same nerve, or nerves which

[10] J. B. Winslow, *Exposition anatomique de la Structure du Corps humain*, Paris, 1732, p. 461.

have been bound by the same membrane at their origin, should sympathize equally with each other, which could not be observed:
. . . if the delirium which generally attends an inflammation of the diaphragm were owing, as has been alledged, to a remote connection between the phrenic and the fifth pair of nerves which sends filaments to the dura mater; why should not an inflammation of the lungs, stomach and intestine, be attended with that symptom as often and in a greater degree, since the fifth pair of nerves hath a more immediate connection with the intercostal than with the phrenic nerves?[11]

Similarly, one would expect the irritation of the fifth pair of nerves in toothache to produce sneezing.

The *involuntary* nature of these actions has made a greater contribution to the history of the sympathetic system than their crude mechanism. Vieussens, for example, described the startled motion of the heart at sudden sounds, and attributed it to the membrane binding the fifth and intercostal pairs of nerves. One can see here a dim perception of an autonomic action, as with the idea of Johnstone (1764) that the ganglia serve to prevent determinations of the will from reaching the viscera. Whytt rejected this mechanism, finding an explanation in the rigidly determined relationship between sentient principle and body.

Since sympathy presupposes feeling, nerves are the mechanism of feeling, and all nerves originate in the brain and spinal marrow, Whytt asserted that all sympathy was to be referred to the brain and spinal marrow; these organs, the principal seat of the soul, were the necessary intermediate structure by which sympathy was effected. This Whytt proved by a repetition of Hales' important experiment on a decapitated and pithed frog: without the substance of its brain and spinal marrow, there was no sympathy between the stimulated toe and the leg muscle which would, in the presence of the spinal cord, retract the toe. Whytt speaks of the 'laws of union between body and soul' and the soul acting as a necessary agent, which makes the above action everything of a reflex; for more complex actions the result depends upon the nature of the stimulus. Thus though the intestine jejunum and rectum both have nervous connections to the diaphragm and both are sensitive, the different nature of the stimulus from the rectum results in a continual sympathetic contraction of the diaphragm, while if the latter is sympathetic to the orifice of the stomach, the contraction is convulsive. The common sensorium is in this way affected differently and hence modifies its influence on the motor organ.

[11] *Works*, p. 508.

Whytt argued that afflictions of the mind produce similar bodily appearances to those of sympathetic origins,[12] and it was thus reasonable to imagine the mind stimulated by sensations of receptor organs could act in the same way. If a nerve of any organ is stimulated, then only that organ is affected, not its sympathetic neighbours; the nerve is one-way, does not affect the brain, and thus is without the influence of sympathy.

Whytt's ideas on the relationship between body and soul will be dealt with in greater detail later. It is sufficient to note here that in sympathy, the soul acts necessarily, unconsciously and on the whole 'wisely'; that is, its actions tend to rid the body of the unpleasant or dangerous stimulus acting upon it. Thus he disagrees with contemporary mechanism in substituting an unknowable soul for an over-simple device of nerves; he borrows from Stahl (if at all) only in having a 'wise' soul, which however is bound by its laws, in action, and is quite unconscious. This is a quasi-mechanism which may be imperfect: the sympathy by which the body reacts in fevers to the unpleasant stimulus in the blood may result in generating motion which the fabric of the body cannot sustain, with fatal results.

Whytt describes three types of 'sympathy' which are not of this nature and are hardly to be considered as true sympathy. First, that due to proximity of parts is nearest to older ideas on sympathy: such may be between the neck of the bladder and the extremity of the rectum; swelling of the face in toothache; vomiting from an inflammation of the liver; inflammation of the cornea and increased sensitivity of the retina, and between the larynx and pharynx. A 'kind of inflammation' may be propagated along the nerves of an inflamed part to its neighbour.

Secondly, a tumour pressing on a nerve will affect the organ at the destination of the nerve. Thirdly, there is often anomalous sympathy in morbid cases, for which Whytt offers no explanation, other than a disordered general sympathy. He gives detailed cases of a girl who coughed when her foot was bent further than a certain angle, and a rash developed from a sprained ankle.

Whytt's normal sympathy was of two types: a general sympathy extending through the body, and a specific sympathy between organs. The 'general sympathy' was due to the almost universal power of sensibility of the various parts of the body; all have

[12] The first on his list of half-a-dozen such changes is increase of the heartbeat in anger, which is still regarded as one of the prime functions of the sympathetic system. The others are: debility from lack of nervous power in fear; blushing in shame; lack of circulation in sadness; (and dull eyes in grief from the same cause) and increased circulation in joy.

nerves and all these lead to the brain; the brain receives all sensations from all over the body and by means of the sentient principle, discharges its motor functions equally everywhere. This general sympathy was not a mechanism of bodily co-ordination as was the specific sympathy, but an 'awareness' of the sensible parts of the body by each other. This would be stimulated into an avoiding action in unusual circumstances. In certain pathological states, for example in the case of the cough upon bending the foot, the (sympathetic) sensibility of the body organs, for instance the lungs, is heightened, and any stimulus, normally ineffective, will throw the lungs and diaphragm into a convulsive effort to rid itself of this stimulus.

Specific sympathy is an extended case of general sympathy. The action of a stimulus upon a sentient principle which necessarily throws into motion the mechanisms best employed to remove the original stimulus is the basis of Whytt's total neuromuscular physiology.

Such specific sympathies are 'wise', as mentioned above. The contraction of the pupil to excess light is such, and was later to become known as 'Whytt's reflex'. Other examples are the contractions of the abdominal muscles in labour and sneezing. He has an extensive list of specific sympathies, some of which would now be regarded as under sympathetic control, some as non-autonomic reflexes and some as hormonal. The stomach is probably the organ of most profound sympathy (also the seat of many nervous disorders), in consent chiefly with the brain (which of course is part of the sympathy of all organs). The uterus has a distinct sympathy with the breasts, and a lesser with other organs.

The prefatory section on sympathy is itself prefixed with an analysis of the structure of the nerves. These, observes Whytt, arise from the medulla of the brain or spine, of which they are continuations. Each anatomical 'nerve' is composed of smaller fibres, and these of yet smaller; the ultimate size of the smallest fibre is not known. All are unbranched from origin to termination.

At this time a physiological dispute of some importance concerned the existence of a fluid in the nerves. The old idea of a subtle fluid moving along the nerves from the brain to inflate the muscles still had its adherents: James Johnstone believed such a mobile spirit moved through, and was redirected by, the ganglia, and by which spirit were generated sensation and motion. Lancisi had thought the ganglia were subsidiary muscles to impel the fluid with greater force, and Dr. Stuart, in 1731, and Burggrav satisfied themselves by means of experiments that the nerves contained a fluid. Whytt is cautious lest he commit himself to an unjustified view:

36

Although it seems probable that the nerves, which are continuations of the medullary substance of the brain and spinal marrow, derive from thence a fluid; yet the extreme smallness of the nervous tube and the subtility of that fluid which they contain, make us altogether ignorant of its peculiar nature and properties. Nor do we know certainly whether this fluid serves only for the support and nourishment of the nerves or whether it be not the medium by which all their actions are performed.[13]

The 'support and nourishment' is unusual; any nervous fluid was commonly thought of as the mechanism of the function of the nerves. Elsewhere[14] Whytt remarks that the extreme exility of the nerves renders it unlikely that they are nourished by a fluid from the brain, and it is probable that they are nourished by blood vessels, in the same way as the brain; for nerves are paralysed by loss of this blood. Whytt was familiar with experiments in which the motion of a muscle could be arrested by a ligature of a blood vessel: that such acted upon the nerve was determined by stimulating the muscle into activity by direct touch.

He is, however, certain that the contraction of muscles is not due to a greater influx of spirits into them. He points out that muscles do not increase in bulk as they contract; that secretion of the nervous fluid must be very slow as the nerves are very small, nor is there any reason to imagine effervescence takes place; that muscles become tendinous in age, which would not occur if they were habitually inflated; that if the cavities in the muscles were cylindrical or spherical, the overall contraction could not be more than one-fifth or one-third respectively of their length, which in the sphincters *pupillae* and *ani* is so; and finally that an excised frog's heart beats far too long for its motion to be explained on the basis of nervous spirit remaining in any segment of nerve, even assuming that such spirit had any reason to move into the muscle.

Thus Whytt does not absolutely deny the existence of a nervous *fluid*—it may exist to keep the nerve fibres fit to be acted upon by the sentient principle—but finds no need to have recourse to the old idea of confusion of *spirits*[15] to explain nervous disorders, and certainly does not believe that any such spirit or fluid acts on the muscles by inflation.[16] He elsewhere speaks of the 'electrical fluids'

[13] *Works*, p. 489.
[14] Ibid., p. 492.
[15] Strictly, animal spirits, The nervous spirits of the eighteenth century were the Galenic animal spirits pursuing their functions in the nerves.
[16] However, he describes this as the common opinion. In another paper he actually calculated the force of the nervous fluid, supposing it to be driven solely by the heart, and thus showed it to be absurdly incapable of inflating muscles.

and 'that subtle fluid', light, so that 'nervous fluid' must not be given too materialistic an interpretation. In general, Whytt observes that if he should speak of 'nervous spirits' he would wish that it should be taken as nothing more than a convenient expression.

In the action of the nerves upon the small vessels, the pulling of the nerve was an alternative theory of nervous action, entertained, Whytt claims, by Vieussens and Willis, whose doctrine of chemical explosion attempted to explain muscle contraction in yet another way. Whytt shows (with Haller) that the nerves are not suitably disposed in their integuments to act as pulling cords, are not muscular, but soft (and therefore unsuitable to transmit vibrations, as another current hypothesis held) and have never been seen to contract. Such action, mechanical or not, would be responsible, for example, for blushing. Duvernoy believed the erection of the penis was owing to the mobility of the nerves constricting the small vessels. Albinus and Whytt argued it was due to increased activity of the small vessels.

So far in this chapter we have discussed the historical background to Whytt's ideas, his normal general sympathy, which is the body's sense of organic unity, and the specific sympathy, which is a normal physiological mechanism. His nervous diseases, then, may be thought of as examples of *pathological* sympathy, general and specific.

He introduces nervous diseases to us as those which were previously known as hypochondriac or hysteric, and this at once suggests a connecting thread which runs through this otherwise tedious compilation of cases and remedies. Hypochondria was the condition in man arising from a disturbed *hypochondre* or gut, and the corresponding disease in women was hysteria, from a disordered uterus. These two organs from classical times had been the seats of the most profound sympathies in the body: the uterus had the clearest relationship to the breasts in the normal working of the body, and in disease it subjected almost every part of the body to a sympathetic suffering. Both organs had important sympathies with the heart, and more notably with the head: both the epilepsy of Galen and the melancholy of the middle ages had recognized sympathetic origins.

For Whytt this pathological sympathy was complicated by other factors. The nerves themselves were likely to suffer diseases of their coats or marrow, and become uncertain in their sensitivity, quantitatively and qualitatively. (Whytt believed that nerves from a sense organ were limited to receive only one kind of stimulus. This could change in disease.) Motor nerves might be excessively feeble, or discharge their function too frequently, as in tetanus. The outcome of all this was a host of symptoms which defied classi-

38

fication: faintings, palpitations, convulsions, vertigo and a large number of alimentary disturbances.

Of this, Whytt makes the best he can. Sufferers from nervous diseases, he said, on the whole fall into two categories, those in otherwise good health whose 'uncommon delicacy' of the nervous system renders them liable to disturbance from any unusual internal or external circumstance, and those with a constant weakness in one or more of the seats of hypochondria or hysteria. Two similar causes acted upon these two kinds of patients, the predisposing, which were not instrumental, but which rendered the sufferer liable to attack by a cause of the second kind, the occasional, that is, the immediate.

The predisposing causes were either an excessive delicacy and sensibility of the whole nervous system, or a weakness or depraved feeling in some organs of the body. The first of these may be an original condition of the body or may be acquired through high or low living, and excessive suffering. The second may be the result of previous illnesses in various organs, or due to sympathy with other organs, most often the stomach and intestines. He gives many examples: a patient who developed a sudden dislike for the smell of coffee, and was prone to sickness upon passing a coffee house; 'Mr. Boyle tells of a nobleman who was apt to faint away when a tansy was brought near him'.[17] He noted the aversion to cats, and Boerhaave's observation that the smell of cheese had been known to occasion bleeding at the nose.

Allied to Whytt's notion of a weakness or depraved function of the nerves of an organ, as a predisposing cause of nervous disorders, was his idea of the specific functions of the nerves. He considered the nerves of different organs to have different 'sensations' arising from these organs and the nature of their function. Thus air produces a satisfactory sensation upon the nerves of the lungs, but causes pain in the stomach, and vice versa with food. In a similar way, the same nerves of one organ may change in time, so that a once agreeable sensation becomes unbearable, as in hydrophobia. Also the same nerves in different people are often subject to different sensations by the same stimulus. Thus, morbid matter in the blood or stimulating medicines will vary considerably in their effects. In his essay on the vital and involuntary motions of animals, Whytt had expressed this as a 'peculiar sensibility' of the nerves; he says ' . . . that which proves a strong stimulus to the nerves of one part will more weakly affect those of another, and vice versa . . . light which by irritating the retina, occasions the contraction of the

17 Ibid., p. 543.

39

pupil, does not act sensibly as a stimulus upon any other part of the body'.[18] Later he says: 'The nerves of different organs in the same animal are so constituted as to be very differently affected even by the same things: so that we cannot absolutely judge by our taste and smell how far any liquor may or may not be adapted to act as a stimulus upon the nerves of a particular organ'.[19]

By the later work of Bell (and Müller) these phenomena became generalized under the heading of the Specific Energies of Nerves: this seems to have been an original observation by Whytt. Carmichael, discussing the matter, says: 'These suggestions of Whytt seem of so definite a nature that it may be that in a previous paper [i.e. of Carmichael] too much assurance was displayed in claiming absolute priority of discovery of this doctrine for Sir Charles Bell'.[20]

The second of Whytt's two categories of causes of nervous diseases was the occasional cause, i.e. that immediately responsible for the disorder. Such causes were to be known as general if their seat was in the blood, and particular if they were to be found in organs.

In both of these Whytt shows his debt to older ideas of sympathy. Galen had insisted upon the uterus as a cause of sympathy: its disordered state from suppression of the menses, or the corruption of retained semen sympathetically affected the brain by way of the sixth pair of nerves, and also generated humours which rose up to the brain, and other organs.[21] These humours are much the same as Whytt's 'morbid matter' which could be generated in the uterus in the same way, and which could descend upon a variety of organs, producing direct disease in them and in others with which they had sympathetic relationships. Other morbid substances in the blood were produced from fevers and skin diseases imprudently checked, or they could be varieties of the wandering gout, which, Whytt believed, could descend upon the stomach with sufficient force to sympathetically stop the heart. Causes within the organs were similar, and usually led to those in the blood: the improper functioning of the viscera produced a general disturbance, as high seasoned meats and strong sauces enervated the stomach, tainted the blood and were likely to breed arthritic matter.

It had long been recognized that almost all sympathizing organs had an important 'consent' to the brain, and the practically

[18] *Essay on the Vital and other Involuntary Motions of Animals*, p. 11.
[19] Ibid., p. 28.
[20] Leonard Carmichael, 'Robert Whytt, a contribution to the history of physiological psychology', *Psychol. Rev.*, 1927, *34*, 287.
[21] Galen, *De affectorum locorum notitiae*, bk. 6, p. xxxviii.

40

invariable companion of hypochondriac diseases were pains in the head or some kind of melancholy. Whytt added to this that the sympathy may be reversed in the pathological states he is discussing, so that a prolonged melancholy might cause hypochondriac diseases and even obstructions of the gut, by 'a fixed spasm'. It is central to Whytt's doctrine that the brain (and spinal cord) is the *fons et origo* of all sympathy, and the importance it thus assumes (greater even than in ancient schemes) in normal physiological sympathy must be expected to appear also in pathological sympathy —nervous diseases. Not only can the brain create hypochondriac diseases, but also 'violent afflictions' of the mind have far-reaching consequences in the body.

Those bodily changes which occur with anger and fear are almost all governed by what is now known as the sympathetic system, and which Whytt explained in terms of sympathy of the brain with each stimulated organ: anger quickens the pulse and respiration, and increases the force (as speed) of the heart. Thus there is an increased flow of saliva due to this heightened circulation; he gives authorities who claim this can also cause anomalous bleeding, at the nipples, for instance. There are bilious vomitings under this condition and a looseness of the bowels under the influence of fear, which, again, produces palpitations and increased beat of the heart, and quickened respiration. The chief functions of the sympathetic nervous system are now recognized to be control of the viscera, and in times of emergency (fear and anger) to increase the rate of general metabolism, according to Cannon's law, so promoting the general activity of the animal: heart-beat is hastened, muscle-tone increased and blood is largely diverted from the gut (which accounts for Whytt's alimentary symptoms) to the muscles and brain. Other hysteric and hypochondriac symptoms may follow from this stoppage of the gut. Whytt notes that women may, in anger, experience a sudden contraction of the bowels, attended by a flatulent or hysteric colic.

Surprise, horror or grief may act in different ways. 'Lord Verulam was wont to faint upon seeing an eclipse',[22] and a woman observing a comet of 1681 was so overcome that she died. Any of the most violent passions are likely to terminate in convulsions, catalepsy, epilepsy, or death. Profound grief often occasions fainting, sometimes in frequent and regular fits.

The phenomenon of hysteric or other fits stimulated in an observer by the sight of one in progress was well known. Whytt mentions that hysteric women in the Royal Infirmary of Edinburgh

[22] *Works*, p. 579.

often promoted general hysteria in this way. Boerhaave made similar observations. Baglivi speaks of a 'young man of Dalmatia' who 'caught' an epileptic fit by observing another. Whytt describes at some length an epidemic disease, known as 'convulsive fits' upon the island of Zetland. The young unmarried women of the island were largely the victims of this disorder, which affected them *en masse*, at public meetings, or in church. (This may be the type of mass hysteria we are more acquainted with now.) Upon the stimulus of preacher or public speaker, the victims developed palpitations of the heart, and fell to the ground 'crying terribly' while the fit lasted, for about fifteen minutes; the legs were alternately extended and withdrawn, and respiration was difficult. Generally those who suffered were more prone to more attacks, but emerged unhurt and were otherwise quite healthy.

Whytt notes that yawning and vomiting are similarly 'infectious', and described it as the 'still more wonderful sympathy' between the nervous systems of different people, 'by impressions made upon the sensorium commune',[23] and acting on the nervous system. Much of this seems to come from his teacher Boerhaave, who in his book on the diseases of the nerves, in the section on 'sympathy', surprisingly makes little mention of visceral control, but is concerned with that of the sensorium, both internally and externally.

It was suggested at the beginning of this section that the nervous diseases which Whytt described were pathological states of sympathy, and that it was by his rationalized scheme of sympathy that his nervous diseases would be examined. Not all pathological sympathies from this viewpoint can be seen to be 'general' and 'specific' as were the normal sympathies (for example that between the *sensoria* of different persons, just described) but many do fall into these two categories.

Thus the normal physiological sympathy whereby the heart, lungs, kidneys, intestines, etc., pursued their functions was this, that the sensitive nerves on the inside of each organ, affected by the presence of the contents of the organ, communicated sympathetically to the sentient principle, and that to the nerves controlling the muscles pertaining to each organ. The result was that the contents of the organs—blood, air, urine, nutriment—were moved on to avoid the disagreeable 'sensation' they had originally occasioned. The blood circulated, air was taken in and expelled and the urine and faeces discharged.

In a pathological state, perhaps directly from the sentient principle in 'prolonged melancholy', or sympathetically from

[23] *Works*, p. 583.

42

damage elsewhere, the sensitivity of the nerves would be altered, resulting in variations of the pulse, asthma, excess or too little urine, and disturbances within the gut. The latter could be produced experimentally in a dog by severing the eighth pair of nerves (i.e. the vagus). This is pathological specific sympathy, a perversion of a normal physiological process.

Disordered general sympathy is exemplified by the case Whytt gives of a girl whose whole nervous system was so unnaturally sensitive that if her foot were turned through a certain angle, she invariably coughed.[24]

How did Whytt deal with all this? His characteristic ingenuity spent itself upon discovering the sympathies which lay at the root of these diseases, and for his treatment of them he relied on the orthodox collection of medicines and practices. He did evolve a medicine for his own disordered stomach, giddiness and faintness, and it became known as 'Whytt's Tincture':

R.Cort.Peruvian Pulv. unc.iv.

Rad.Gentian.

Cort. Aurant.ana.unc.i. ss. Misc.

Infunde in spir. vin. Gall.in balneo arenae per dies vi et eola.

Whytt took one tablespoon twice a day.

He tackled each of the causes of the disorders in recognized ways. Weakness of the nervous system, a predisposing cause and a precursor to pathological general and specific sympathies, if arising from causes other than the original constitution of the body, must be strengthened by the use of bitters: gentian root, *cortices aurantiorum* and *summitates centaurii minoris* taken in wine. Steel and iron waters were also commonly used as strengthening medicines, both in their artificial form and as mineral waters, the chalybeates of Bath and Pyrmont. Inherent and excessive sensibility of the nervous system could only be treated with remedies which lessened that sensibility, like opium, which, Whytt insisted, acted upon the extremities of the nerves, or by means of the pediluvium and semi-cupium, which relax the body. Such remedies are short term, allowing the body to recover naturally from the condition to which its sensibility has led it.

Morbid matter and acrid humours may, by the uncertainty of their action, be described also as causes of disordered general sympathy.

[24] 'In my Opinion,' wrote a disgruntled medical student, having made his way through Whytt's long and rather tedious observations, 'Dr. Whytt has been a Dancing Master before he practic'd Physick otherwise he would never have put this poor Girl in 24 different positions for (as I think) his own amusement—he has exceeded the celebrated French Dancing Master La Glasse by 6 Positions.' (Marginalia from a copy of the *Works* in Edinburgh University Library, p. 160.)

They were treated by medicines which caused them to be thrown out of the body as eruptions or with the excreta, or by those which prevented their formation. Of this sort is the wandering gout, which is treated with bark and bitters. The 'scorbutic' matter which was the cause of *lepra Graecorum* and tetters could be driven to the surface by vomits, warm stomachics and sudorifics, and cured by 'mild mercurials'.

Specific pathological sympathies were treated in the same way, with medicaments proper to their nerves and constitution. Such short-term treatments should be followed by strengthening medicines and long-term beneficial activities. Whytt pays considerable attention to diet, warns against intemperance of any sort, and strongly advocates exercise. Bathing in the sea was medically if not fashionably recognized (Sir John Floyer had written a *History of Cold Bathing* and 'Brighthelmstone' was known for its curative water), and if Gilchrist of Dumfries recommended sailing, then Whytt was not backward in his advocacy of horse riding.[25]

Lastly, those nervous diseases which proceeded from violent affections of the mind were treated at their origin. To arrest the attention of a wandering *sensorium* was often to disperse the symptoms its errant sensibilities occasioned. There were several ways of doing this: acrid cataplasms competed in medical preferences with artificially-created blisters; dry cupping and friction all strove to divert the affected mind with a greater pain and thus concentrate its diverse and pathological sympathies. 'A greater pain destroys a lesser' was a dictum of Hippocrates well known to Whytt, and he gives examples of sufferers cured by its application: a hydrophobic enabled to drink water after a cold bath, and the cure of epileptics by whipping. A French girl in 1752 seems to have been cured of the same complaint by the firing of a gun at her bedside as she recovered from a fit.

Little emerges from this paper of Whytt's except his use of a rationalized system of sympathy. It is essentially a practical treatise, full of observations and recommendations, but on the theoretical side seems to have played a large part in concentrating attention on the part played by the nerves in the well-recognized diseases of hysteria and hypochondria ('hyp').

In this way it characterized, if it did not cause the decline of an aspect of humoral pathology. Books before this dealt with vapours and movements of humours from the spleen, usually associated with a greater or lesser degree of mechanism. Whytt opposed all this, and seems indirectly to have started a fashion for fits of 'nerves' rather

[25] *Works*, p. 633.

than fits of the 'vapours'. This is described in a later chapter. Perhaps the French translation of the book fulfilled a similar function, but Haller's summary of it was marked by caution. He noted as its important points (whether or not he agreed with them) the following: sympathy does not depend on connections between branches of nerves; affections of the mind are associated with oscillations of the small vessels; hypochondriac diseases can develop from a lessened sensibility of the nerves; inflammation is produced by a spasmodic contraction of the small blood vessels; and bones, cartilage and the dura mater are sensible. Of these, Whytt's observations on sympathy and the part played by the mind might now be considered more important. Whytt's recognition of the extent to which emotional factors 'penetrate into or become an integral factor in the pathogenesis of clinical disorders is exemplary and modern'.[26]

[26] Editorial article, *J. Am. med. Ass.*, 1964, *189*, 150.

CHAPTER V

Smaller Works

Whytt's remaining works include two important essays, the second of his *Physiological Essays*, on sensibility and irritability, and the treatise on vital and involuntary motions, both of which will be considered later. This chapter is concerned with a number of smaller papers distributed through various journals.

1. An Account of the Earthquake felt at Glasgow and Dumbarton; also of a Shower of Dust falling on a Ship between Shetland and Iceland

This paper is part of a letter to Sir John Pringle, and was read on 19 February 1756 to the Royal Society and published in the *Philosophical Transactions*, 1755–6, *49*, part 2, 509. The paper is very short and describes the events concisely. The ship in question was voyaging from Leith to Charles-town in South Carolina: Whytt may have had some connection with this part of the American colonies, as his correspondent, Dr. Lining, was a resident of that area. The dust, concluded Whytt, derived from the eruption of Hecla in Iceland.

There was a large seismic disturbance in the winter[1] of 1755–56; there are at least a dozen papers in the *Philosophical Transactions* of that year recording tide irregularities in the Thames, and similar disturbances over a wide area. The earliest seems to be a report from America in the October, with others following from Britain and Switzerland, Leyden, Brussels, Antigua and Maestricht, up to the following February.

2. The Use of Sublimate in the Cure of Ulcers

The collected works of 1768 include extracts of Whytt's correspondence on the subject of ulcers. The first is from a letter to Pringle dated 15 January 1757, in which he describes several cases of 'carcinomatous or phagedaenic' ulcers which he cured by Baron van Swieten's medicine for the lues venera, i.e. corrosive sublimate in malt spirits. The sores were washed externally with the medicine, which was also taken internally.

---

[1] Lisbon was destroyed by an earthquake on 1 November 1755. In the *Essays and Observations, Physical and Literary* of Edinburgh there are various papers on disturbances in Loch Ness, Loch Lomond, the Firth of Forth, and Closeburn Loch, and one on the Earthquake at Dumbarton.

Pringle replied, shortly after, that 'phagedaenic' was of 'vague signification'. Whytt wrote back on 17 March with two cases, of a 'carcinomatous' ulcer of the cheek and nose and a scorbutic ulcer of the leg, both of which he cured by the use of the corrosive sublimate. He also describes a case of a 'kind of cancerous ulcer of the nose'. The patient had been unsuccessfully treated with mercury pills from the Edinburgh Dispensary, yet Whytt achieved moderate success with the sublimate. The sore was also known as *herpes exedens, nome, noli me tangere* or *ulcus depascens*. Internal use of the sublimate was also required to rid the blood of the morbid matter.

There is also a letter from a Mr. Spottiswood to Whytt, vouching for the cure of one of Whytt's cases.

3. An Account of the Electrical Virtue in a Cure of the Palsy

This paper[2] was read to the Royal Society in December 1757, having been sent to the Secretary, the Rev. Thomas Birch, D.D., by Pringle.

The cure was performed by a Patrick Brydone upon Elizabeth Foster. She had, about 1742, been seized with a violent nervous fever, giving rise to asthma and general weakness. In 1755 she had the fever again, which resulted this time in the paralysis of the limbs of the left side, which yet remained sensible. Although better in the warm weather, she later lost this sensibility as well. The administering of six hundred severe shocks in three days apparently effected a 'complete cure'.

4. An Account of an Epidemic Distemper in Edinburgh and several Other Parts in the South of Scotland in the Autumn of 1758

This paper, published in *Medical Observations and Enquiries*, vol. 11,[3] first appeared in a letter to Pringle dated 10 November 1758.

Whytt observed that at the time of the epidemic, the weather was dry and mild, there having been an easterly wind during most of the summer. In the July and August there had been a 'fever with a bloody flux' in Argyl, Newcastle, and an area a dozen miles south of Edinburgh. In September and October there had been a small outbreak of smallpox in Edinburgh, severe in Teviotdale and Coupar.

The epidemic itself ran from 20 September to 24 October, and moved across the country from the east. Seven out of every eight suffered, and in the Carse of Gowrie the horses also fell victims to the affliction.

Whytt described the symptoms. People were differently afflicted,

[2] Published in the *Works* of 1768.
[3] This reference is from R. Watt, *Bibliotheca Britannica*, Edinburgh, 1827, vol. 2, p. 966. The paper is also in the *Works*.

47

but the disease generally began with a sore throat and feverishness, followed by a cough. There was a headache in the forehead, and watery eyes. If there was sneezing or discharge at the nose, the fever was not so pronounced; sometimes there was a hard dry cough without a sore throat. Some patients bled at the nose.

Camphire, the sacred tincture, and laudanum had no effect, but sudorific boluses often provided some relief. Whytt suspected a rheumatic humour to be the cause, as in one case the pain moved from the head into the groin and then disappeared. In two cases that he examined, the cough appeared to be critical; the pulse returned to normal after a bout. The morbid matter, Whytt explained, was thrown upon the throat. The fever was not associated with coldness and shivering. In general it seemed to be infectious rather than contagious.

The cure was to keep the patient in bed in the early stages, keeping the body open with clysters and promoting sweat with hot drinks. The fever required bleeding. Few cases resulted in death; if ignored the humour fell upon the lungs and was to be moved by blisters and bleeding.

5. Cases of the Remarkable Effects of Blisters in lessening the Quickness of the Pulse in Coughs, attended by Infarction of the Lungs, and Fever[4]

Blisters were thought to evacuate chiefly the serous humours, while issues and setons discharged purulent matter. Their normal action was to increase the pulse by local inflammation, 'the few particles of the cantharides' entering the blood and stimulating the heart. Whytt noticed, however, that this was not always the case in fevers, which doctors had always been careful of treating with blisters. He described several cases. In the first there was a bad cough, oppression of stomach and breast, a pain in the right side and a pulse of one hundred. The blood was sizy. Whytt applied a blister to the right side, and on the following day the pulse had dropped to 88 and the following day 78. When the blister dried, the pulse rose again to 96, but returned to 72 upon the application of a second blister: the cure was completed.

The second patient had imprudently exposed himself to cold, and had lain for a fortnight with a fever before Whytt was called. The pulse was 112, the patient emaciated and sweating. He produced a thick purulent phlegm. A blister lessened the pulse and cough, which returned upon its drying up. A second blister returned the pulse to 96 and a slow cure began.

He describes two more cases with similar histories, and concludes that the treatment should not be used in 'true peripneumony'

[4] Published in the *Works*, and in *Phil. Trans.*, 1757-8, *50*, 569.

where the lungs are inflamed and bleeding is the proper remedy, but when there is a quantity of phlegm, and the pulse, though quick, is small. In any case, blisters affect pleurisies more than true peripneumonies because the site of pleurisy shares the blood supply of the thorax, where the blister is applied.

In a letter to Pringle on this subject, added at the foot of the paper, Whytt notes that blisters are of no use when the fever proceeds from a malfunction of the brain.

6. Of the Use of the Bark in Dysenteries and a Hoarseness after the Measles[5].

This paper is very short. Whytt observes that the bark was becoming more widely used for an increasing number of maladies and speculates (he does not say why) on its possible use in dysentery. He describes several cases in which he experimented with the use of the medicine and was gratified to find his ideas justified. In several other cases, he found the bark to be of use in curing a hoarseness consequent upon an attack of measles, but owned that this seemed to be its sole use in such convalescents.

7. Observations on the Anomalous and True Gout

The paper before Whytt's in the same edition of *Essays and Observations, Physical and Literary* is by Dr. David Clerk: 'Observations on the Arthritis anomala, with a postscript relating chiefly to the cure of the regular gout', and the actual title of Whytt's paper is 'Some observations on the same subject'.

The paper is again very short, as Whytt claims to be 'unfit' to comment or to criticize Clerk's paper, his thoughts on the matter some while ago having been largely in agreement with Clerk's. He observes that gout had only 'recently' been used to explain some nervous disorders. His only comments upon Clerk's paper are that he was uncertain of the value of tansy in treating the gout, and that he had himself to stop taking cicuta (for another disorder) as it increased his flatulence, and 'faintness at the stomach' which he knew to be caused by gout.

Clerk defines true gout as that of the extremities, often associated with age, while that of other parts of the body is anomalous, and is more common than realized, occurring often in young people. Whytt agrees, mentioning that some of his patients had been thirteen or fourteen years old. Clerk defines *Arthritis anomala imperfecta* as that which moves from parts of the body to the extremities, and *Arthritis anomala perfecta* as that with the opposite tendency. Much of this seems to derive from Musgrave.

[5] *Essays and Observations, Physical and Literary*, 1771, 3, 366.

49

8. A Description of the Matrix or Ovary of the Buccinum Ampullatum

This paper was published in the Edinburgh *Essays and Observations, Physical and Literary*, 1756, *2*, 8, and the second edition of 1771. The specimen was sent to Whytt by Dr. Alexander Garden of New York, and seems to be the fruit of an exotic plant which was occasionally washed up on the shore of that part of the American Colonies and sometimes mistaken by the inhabitants for the hardened froth of the sea. The paper is little more than an annotated diagram.

9. An Account of some Experiments made with Opium on living and dying Animals

This paper appears in the *Works* of 1768, and in the *Essays and Observations, Physical and Literary*, 1756, *2*, 280.

Opium was a well-known and powerful drug of recognized properties: Whytt's old teacher Young had lectured on it, and it formed a major part of Whytt's treatment of nervous disorders. Experiments to determine the method of its action were not uncommon; the ancients thought it to work by reason of its excessive cold, and later it was thought to be a heating medicine (e.g. Alston),[6] rarefying the blood and compressing the brain. Observations of the distended veins of opiated animals may have lent support to this theory, but Whytt argued this was a result of the slowing of the heart. He also was aware, however, of Alston's observation that circulation stopped first in the small vessels, which would concentrate the blood in the arteries.

Whytt believed that the action of opium was upon the extremities of the nerves of the part to which it was applied. At such points, it simply lessened the power of the nerve: those admitting sensation to the *sensorium commune* were less efficient, and those controlling muscular motion produced diminished contraction. This action was direct: the opium did not send 'effluvia' into the blood, or dissolve in it that it should be carried to the nervous system or muscles. Whytt satisfied himself upon this last count by injecting opium into the stomach and gut of two frogs. From one he removed the heart, and observed that it was 'quite dead' in half an hour, yet having no circulation to disseminate the opium. The other, intact, still had a pulse of seventeen per minute after an hour. To ensure that it was not simply the removal of the heart that killed the first frog, Whytt performed the same operation upon a non-opiated frog, which continued to jump for one hour and remained alive for two and a half.

Such a viewpoint was not uncommon; Doctors Jones, Alston, Van Swieten and Boerhaave also believed opium acted upon

[6] C. Alston, 'A dissertation on opium', *Edinburgh Medical Essays*, 1746, *1*, 132.

the nerves of the area to which it was applied, did not enter the blood, and acted upon the rest of the nervous system by sympathy. Dr. Jones in fact (*Mysteries of Opium Revealed*)[7] accepted that a negligible quantity entered the blood, and Willis and Van Swieten thought that the extraordinary sympathy of the stomach accounted for the effects of opium received there.

Whytt, without mentioning sympathy, was in a similar position. Having shown opium is not distributed by the blood, he demonstrated that its effects are broadcast by the brain and nerves: he took two frogs and decapitated the first, destroying also the spinal marrow. From both he stripped an area of skin from the abdomen, and bathed them in opium. After half an hour the heart of the whole frog was beating only six times a minute, while that of its decapitated partner was still beating at eighteen after an hour, and at sixteen after another threequarters of an hour. Possibly Whytt was not content to refer the action of opium via the nerves upon the remainder of the nervous system to sympathy, as he noted that opium taken into the stomach, an organ of the most widespread sympathy, acted less quickly than that introduced into the body cavities. Langrish experimented with laurel water, with similar results.

Monro, writing later, disagrees with Whytt in general in believing that opium did in fact enter the blood, and, in particular, over this experiment. Whytt merits his usual judgement as 'ingenious': 'Before that time [i.e. 1756] and more fully since, Dr. Whytt has endeavoured to prove several particulars respecting the manner in which opium affects animals, by a variety of ingenious experiments, some of which are much more decisive than any formerly proposed'.[8]

But, added Monro, Whytt was incorrect in this instance: the effect of destroying the brain and spinal marrow was to slow the heartbeat, and hence it would lessen the absorption of and distribution of opium by the blood.

Monro's criticism is not entirely borne out by a close examination of the two experiments in question, particularly as in the immediately previous experiment, Whytt pithed a frog whose heart subsequently beat at a greater rate than either of the others for over nine hours. Whytt offered as further proof that opium acts on the nerves and probably the medulla cerebri, an experiment of Alston, who injected opium into the crural vein of a dog, and observed its rapid demise.

[7] From Alexander Monro, 'How opium . . . acts on nerves to which it is applied and brings the rest of the nervous system into sufference by sympathy', *Essays and Observations, Physical and Literary*, 1771, *3*, 296.

[8] Ibid.

He also argues that the action of opium is too rapid to be explained by its distribution in the blood, a point ignored by Monro. Whytt uses as an example the dog which almost immediately lost the use of its legs. Similarly there could be no time for physical 'effluvia' to act on the central nervous system by way of the nerves.

Whytt believed that this action of opium was general throughout the body: it universally destroyed the power of feeling and motion, and acted more quickly in those animals whose parts do not live long without each other and which are readily killed by want of air and food. Dogs, in Whytt's example, are more susceptible than frogs; he quotes two experiments by Robert Ramsay, who injected opium into the rectum and abdomen of a dog, which lost the power of its limbs 'almost instantly' and one by Mead, who introduced the drug into the stomach of a dog.

Haller disagreed with Whytt: 'Opium does not act from without directly upon the nerves; the results of new experiments by Fontana and Caldani are contrary with Whytt's doctrine'.[9] He also[10] denied that opium had an effect upon the heart. By a number of experiments, Whytt satisfied himself that his idea was correct: the heart is stopped, like other muscles, but not so quickly. These experiments involved non-opiated pithed frogs whose hearts continued to beat longer than whole frogs treated with opium, and frogs' excised hearts which beat much longer and faster in water than in opium solution. Clearly the loss of the nervous system was not such a bar to the motion of the heart as the effects of opium at that place or propagated by the nerves. Haller's opinion sprang from his great physiological premise: irritability (i.e. contractility) was an inherent power of the muscular 'glue', and could act independently of the influence of the nerves. A ligature upon a nerve, he argued, still left the muscle with the ability to contract. In this paper, Whytt put forward this defence of his ideas, that opium acts more intimately than a ligature (which allows nervous influence to remain below it) and prevents voluntary motion and irritability, which are immediately dependent upon the influence of the nerves, by acting upon the extremities of these nerves, *before* it was able to reach the muscles. It was over this point that Whytt and Haller chiefly differed. Haller accepted that opium in some way reduced muscular action and Whytt admitted that opium, having reached

[9] A. von Haller, *Elementa Physiologiae Corporis Humanae*, Lausanne, 1757-66, vol. 5, p. 605. He quotes Whytt more often than most writers on opium, and discusses his ideas in relation to those of Berger, Alston, Borrich and Smellie (who once dreamed that Whytt and Monro settled a medical dispute by means of cudgels) among others.

[10] *Act. Götting.*, 2, 147. From Whytt's *Works*, p. 299.

the muscles, might act directly upon them, although he stresses the importance of the neuromuscular junction: 'Its influence reaches to the fibres of the muscles themselves, or to the extremities of the nervous filaments which terminate in them';[11] but he reaffirms that irritability is always dependent on the presence and influence of the nerves. In the section on the reflex action, it will be argued that Whytt was the first to publish that only a segment of the spine was necessary for the maintenance of some involuntary motions. In this paper he noted, from Ramsay's experiments, performed at Whytt's request, that that section of the cord (the inferior) was first affected by opium, while the other motions remained. Whytt concluded that opium does not produce sleep, nor are its actions due to sleep, which may, however, follow as a result of the lessened sensibility of the nerves.

10. *Of the Difference between Respiration and the Motion of the Heart in Sleeping and Waking Persons*

This paper was published in the *Works* of 1768, and in the *Essays and Observations, Physical and Literary*, 1771, *I*, 493. It is an example of Whytt's particular physiology.

The effect of sleep is to render all parts of the body less sensitive by a diminished sensibility of their nerves. Thus the heart, receiving blood more gently from the unused voluntary muscles ('It is well known . . . that the action of the muscles of voluntary motion not only promotes the return of blood to the heart, but determines it thither with much greater force than usual'),[12] becomes much more full than usual before the *stimulus* of the blood excites the heart into contraction. This stimulus is basic to Whytt's doctrine of bodily action: it acts, via the nerves and sentient principle, upon an organ, which reacts in a way generally resulting in the removal of the stimulus. Thus the heart throws out its blood, depending for its speed upon its own sensitivity and the stimulating nature of the blood: acrid humours in disease, increased force in exercise, or higher temperature, are all stimuli. In sleep, quiescence of mind and the prone position render the blood slow and the heart less sensible.

The decreased circulation moves less blood into the lungs. The blood needs less air in relation to its quantity, and the lungs are less sensitive. Thus the stimulus of blood in the lungs is smaller and acts less often upon the lungs, which excite the diaphragm and chest into the motion of inspiration to relieve the situation.

11. In the library of the Royal College of Physicians, Edinburgh, is a collection of some manuscript notes taken by Whytt from the

[11] *Works*, p. 325.
[12] Ibid., p. 179

lectures of George Young, and some notes taken by William Falconer from Whytt's clinical lectures. The latter are largely abbreviated versions of his written works, including hysteric and hypochondriac diseases, dropsies, the use of blisters and pediluvia in fevers, and the nervous atrophy. They are dated 3 December 1762. The former show Whytt's interest in problems of muscular motion and sensation, and some account is given of them in the section below, on the soul.

12. Seller and Watt give false references to papers of Whytt's. Seller mentions a paper on nerve anatomy in the *Essays and Observations, Physical and Literary* which does not appear there, and Watt's reference for 'The Cure of a fractured Tendo Achillis' in the same publication is in fact applicable to a paper by Alexander Monro.

13. *Of the Anthelmintic Virtues of the Root of the Indian Pink, being part of a letter from Dr. John Lining, Physician at Charlestown in South Carolina to Dr. Robert Whytt, Professor of Medicine in the University of Edinburgh*

The title of this paper is self-explanatory. It appears in the *Edinburgh Essays, Physical and Literary* 1754.

14. *An Enquiry into the Causes which promote Circulation of Fluids in the small vessels of Animals*

This is the first of Whytt's *Physiological Essays* which he published in 1755. As described, there was another edition in 1761 and the third, first published in 1766, is included in the *Works* of 1768. It was translated into French by Thébault in 1759 and printed in Paris. It ranks as one of Whytt's more important papers, being derived from his doctrine of involuntary motion: a stimulus acts upon the 'sentient principle' by way of nerves, which itself reacts in an inherent way to rid the body of the (generally unpleasant) stimulus. The first part of the paper is given over to demonstrating that the force of the heart is insufficient to explain total circulation, and particularly that of the capillaries, and the second part to Whytt's explanation of the finer circulation.

The first Harveians thought that the heart accounted for the total circulation, but a lack of knowledge of the microscopic anatomy of the capillaries rendered the matter doubtful. Harvey spoke of 'pores of the flesh', and Borelli believed the small vessels ended in a porous substance, and supposed the blood to enter it as a sponge, 'by gravity' as Whytt explains. Whytt himself was not clear on this point. Hoffman had claimed that blood moved more quickly in the capillaries, but Whytt insists that friction and 'mutual

54

cohesion' of the parts of the blood renders this hypothesis nugatory, and makes clear that the heart and large arteries cannot be solely responsible for circulation.

Whytt proceeds to prove his point mathematically. Stephen Hales had shown, in 1732, from several experiments of a very direct nature on horses, that the force of the heart was equivalent to maintaining a column of blood ninety inches high [13] at the point of entry into the aorta. Thus for any artery, in Whytt's words, 'The momentum of this fluid will be found by multiplying the area of the transverse section of the artery into 90 . . . for the product gives us the number of cubic inches of blood whose weight is equal to the pressing power with which the blood is driven by the force of the heart into the artery.'[14]

If for 'momentum' we read 'destruction of momentum', then this argument becomes intelligible to a modern physicist. Borelli talked of a *vis percussionis*, which, it seemed to be the general opinion, was greater than any finite quiescent resistance (i.e. circulation) and which may have been true momentum, but Whytt's meaning of 'momentum' is not clear. In distinction to Borelli he argues that the force of the heart is a pressing force (Haller considered this was one of the more important points of Whytt's paper) but elsewhere seems to equate this with a 'projectile' force, which has more of true momentum in it: ' . . . or, which is the same thing, that the left ventricle of the heart, does not, by its direct projectile force at every contraction, move forwards the whole circulating fluids in all the vessels of the body.'[15] His calculations certainly show that he thought of momentum as a projectile force, as he speaks of it as the square of the velocity, and as mentioned above and treated of below, his calculations of the force of blood in arteries of different diameters holds good if the energy from the destruction of momentum is treated as the pressing force to sustain a column of blood.

A projectile force is of course rapidly diminished by friction, an argument used by Whytt to explain the need of capillary participation, and it is difficult to see why the idea of relatively slowly moving blood under relatively high pressure, more or less constant during the systole of the heart, was not acceptable.

In order to discover the 'momentum' of the blood in various arteries and the capillaries, Whytt arrives at the general formula above, and a diameter for the latter. Martine, from Leeuwenhoek

[13] The systolic blood pressure in the carotid of man is 90 mm. of mercury, or 48 inches of water.

[14] *Works*, p. 213.

[15] Ibid., p. 218.

and Jurin, believed the red corpuscles of the blood to be 1/1933.5 of an inch.[16] For ease of calculation, Whytt uses 1/2000 (the actual size of a human red corpuscle is 7.5 to 8μ, or approximately 1/3100 of an inch). Since Leeuwenhoek had seen corpuscles bending to get through capillaries, Whytt uses this figure as the effective diameter: the area of cross section will be 0.000,000,196 of an inch. Thus the momentum will be this multiplied by 90, representing the number of inches of blood which would be supported by that momentum, or expressed in weight, 1/214 of a grain. Here momentum is a constant weight dependent on area: it is in fact pressure, and implies something of energy produced by the destruction of momentum. Whytt's calculation is approximately correct, allowing that blood does in fact have a different density from water. Momentum is mass × velocity. The mass of blood is $e\,Av$, where e is density and Av is volume of blood (area × velocity) moving at a given speed. The 'momentum' of blood maintaining a column of 90 inches is, say, a force F. Then $F = e\,Av^2$. Allowing blood to have a density of 1, then 'momentum' is the square of velocity in a capillary of any given area, as Whytt has it elsewhere, and represents the destruction of momentum. Since F is 90 $A\,e$, then rate of destruction of momentum is 90 A, which Whytt uses in his calculations. As mentioned above, a pressure system would not depend upon velocity and thus would not be diminished by friction.

According to Keill the combined volumes of the capillaries was greater than that of the aorta,[17] and the velocity of blood flowing from the latter into the former will decrease. Its velocity in a capillary of 1/2000 of an inch should be, to its velocity in the aorta, as 1 to 345. Thus, adds Whytt, its momentum will be $345^2 = 119,025$. This diminishes Whytt's figure of momentum by a commensurate amount: $(1/214) \times (1/119,025) = 1/25,471,350$ part of a grain. He estimates the weight of a corpuscle as 1/50,000,000 of a grain, so that the 'momentum, or pressing force of such a globule in its capillary artery, arising from the impulsion of the heart, does not exceed twice its own weight'.[18]

Such momentum is further decreased by friction: the velocity of water entering pipes of different diameters with the same force are 'pretty nearly as the square roots of their respective diameters' (Robinson's *Animal OEconomy*, prop. 1, exp. 2).[19] Thus in a capillary

[16] *Edinburgh Medical Essays*, 2, article 7 (from Whytt's *Works*, p. 214). Haller thought the red corpuscle was between 1/2000 and 1/3000 of an inch.

[17] Modern calculations suggest the combined cross sectional area of the capillary bed is about 1000 times that of the aorta.

[18] *Works*, p. 127.

[19] Ibid.

of 1/2000 of an inch arising directly from the aorta, the velocity of blood would be in the proportion of $\sqrt{(2/0.0005)}$ to $\sqrt{(2/0.07)}$: the momentum of a single particle would be as 1 to 1398. The length of the tube also decreases velocity by friction. Hales observed that blood moves 43 times as quickly in the capillary artery of the lung of a frog as in a capillary of the abdomen. Thus, in Whytt's words: 'whether we suppose animal heat to arise from the friction of the blood on the side of the vessel, or from an intestine motion, that *caeteris paribus*, more heat must be generated in the heart and lungs than anywhere else; and hence the necessity of continual supplies of fresh air to cool the blood in its passage through the pulmonary vessels'.[20] Whytt found by experiment that the temperature under the wing of a jackdaw was 104°F; in the rectum 107½°F and 109°F at the heart. A pigeon revealed a similar condition.

Although Hales and Leeuwenhoek had observed an acceleration of the blood in the capillaries at every systole, Whytt argues that the projectile force of the heart, although possibly reaching here, did not cause this.[21] Hales also thought the velocity of blood in the capillaries of the frog to be 900 times slower than in the aorta of man, or two to six times less than Whytt had computed it to be in the human capillary. In such a case: 'Wherefore the excess of momentum of a red globule in such an artery of a frog, above the resistance it had to overcome, only amounted to 1/173,340,000 of a grain'[22] (that is, about a third of its weight).

It is interesting to note that Whytt, often represented as a confirmed animist and even a Stahlian, attempts to disprove a mechanical theory by the use of mathematics. In this paper, assuming for the purposes of argument that the nerves are tubes, he extends his method of computing momentum to discover with what force any nervous fluid could be propelled down the nerves. The tacit conclusion is that the momentum of this is so small that muscle contraction by inflation is quite impossible and neural control by the movement of nervous fluid is unlikely. Porterfield, in the *Edinburgh Medical Essays* (volume 4)[23] had computed the diameter of a single nerve to be 1/210,000 of an inch (this from an experiment of Hook's). If the nerves are indeed tubes (Whytt mentions that Leeuwenhoek 'pretended' to see cavities in the nerves) then their cavities cannot be greater than 1/200,000 of an inch. However, gold can be beaten to a thickness of 1/12,000,000

[20] Ibid., p. 218.
[21] The pulse actually reaches the arterioles, but not the capillaries, an anatomical distinction of which medicine of the time was unaware.
[22] *Works*, p. 220.
[23] Ibid.

of an inch and Newton calculated the thickness of solution in a soap bubble to be 1/3,000,000 of an inch, so such a structure would not be outside the bounds of possibility.

Using similar calculations, Whytt estimates that the moving force behind a globe of animal spirits in a nerve would be only one-nineteenth of its weight.

'Having shown how inconsiderable the *momentum* of the fluids arising from the projectile force of the heart must be . . .',[24] Whytt goes on to consider the insufficiency of the heart from another aspect: the obstacles it must overcome if it were solely responsible for circulation. Borelli computed this resistance of blood to be equal to 180,000 lb., and Whytt, while admitting this is too great, still expresses the resistance in pounds, and thought it more than could be moved by the 51 lb. of which Stephen Hales had calculated the human heart was capable. If such a resistance were due to friction, then it would increase with the velocity and mass of blood. It is difficult to see why it should be expressed as a constant figure, in weight.

The 51 lb. exerted by the heart, according to Hales (Whytt thinks 60 a more likely figure) is over the internal surface of the ventricle, an area of some 15 square inches. Whytt estimates the area of a cross section of the aorta to be approximately half a square inch; the ratio of pressures is then 30:1: 'Hence a resistance in the aorta equal to two pounds will require a force of above 60 lbs. exerted by the whole internal surface of the left ventricle . . .'.[25]

Keill was of the opinion that only a small force is necessary to keep the blood in circulation when it has once started. Whytt argues that in syncope the heart may stop, yet successfully restart. Further, Hales showed that blood returning to the heart has only a tenth of the force which propelled it into the aorta, and thus it is clear that it gains nine-tenths of its force in passing through the heart and lungs. (It was believed that the lungs contributed directly to the pressure of the blood.)

Whytt concluded from all these investigations that the heart had not enough power to account for the whole process of circulation, as its 'projectile force' did not reach the smallest vessels (which thus had no alternate motion). The alternating contraction and dilatation of the large vessels, on the other hand, was due only to the pulse.[26]

In place of those theories which attributed to the heart alone the power of circulating the blood, Whytt sets up his own hypothesis:

[24],[25] Ibid., p. 223.
[26] There is little doubt that the capillaries do vary greatly in volume by their own power, but the significance of this in circulation is uncertain.

the blood, by reason of its composition, heat, and intestine motion, acts as a *stimulus* on the capillaries, and excites them into rapid alternate contractions, or oscillations, by which means the blood is propelled through them at greater velocity. Blood may possess acrid or saline properties, and its heat and motion may throw such particles into greater motion and increase their stimulating nature. Heat is not the least in this; Harvey had shown that the hearts of some shellfish beat only in the warm weather. In the same way does the food excite the gut into motion, and, Whytt adds, the blood in the vena cava. That the small vessels may be responsible for circulation is shown by the existence of animals without hearts and the occasional appearance of monsters without hearts (Van Swieten, *Histoire de l'Académie des Sciences*, 1704, and *Mémoires*, 1740).[27] De Gorter had supposed, like Whytt, that an oscillation of the capillaries was a necessary adjunct to the motion of the heart, and Baglivi had postulated oscillations of vessels,[28] and of membranes, which latter he supposed to derive from movements of the dura mater.

Whytt uses his own revised theory of inflammation to support his doctrine of capillary circulation. The mechanism of inflammation which Whytt opposed was that which suggested inflammation to be due to local contraction of the small vessels with increased force of the heart, so that blood passed through them more vigorously. Whytt argues that, for example, steam or hot spirits of wine causes tears and inflammation without increase in the force of the heart; the action is directly upon the small vessels, which are excited by the acrid vapours into greater oscillations.[29] Blushing, salivating, and the production of pale urine in excess by hysterical women are examples of small vessels locally stimulated by the action of the mind, and owing nothing to increased force of the heart.

That such sensitivity of the small vessels is due to nerves is inherent rather than expressed in this paper. Whytt only particularizes in the case of an arm palsied through lack of nervous power, which shrivelled, as its circulation was much reduced. In the second of the *Physiological Essays* Whytt observes that although

[27] Whytt, *Works*, p. 299.

[28] Modern physiology shows that all the capillaries are invested with nerves of the sympathetic system, and that local skin irritation causes 'axon reflexes', i.e. those which do not reach the spinal cord. That is, as Whytt said, stimuli act directly upon the vessels. The nervous control of blood vessels was not formulated until 1852 by Bernard.

[29] The pulse may become greater in inflammations, by sympathy of the parts, and a blister may lessen an inflammation by its painful sensation destroying the lesser pain of the inflammation.

nerves cannot be traced to small vessels, they must be there as such vessels are painful in inflammations, which are due to oscillations, to which muscle and therefore nerve is a necessary prerequisite.

The motion of blood in capillaries was observed by Leeuwenhoek and Haller as an irregular backwards and forwards motion, which continues when the heart is removed. Although this seems to be owing to oscillations of the capillary wall (as no such motion is seen in blood enclosed in a rigid glass tube) yet no oscillation can be seen. Whytt argues that such a motion may be in extent only 1/150 of the diameter of the capillary; that is, of a vessel 1/2000 of an inch, it will be 1/300,000, and for one wall of this vessel, half that, which would be quite unnoticeable under the microscope. Haller pointed out that this oscillation was a major point in Whytt's essay, but was himself inclined to be sceptical, on account of its small extent. Such a motion would result in very slow progress of a corpuscle, but Hales measured the velocity of one in an abdominal capillary of a frog as an inch in a minute and a half, and Leeuwenhoek and Senac were also of the opinion that such movement was slow. Haller had seen blood moving faster in a mesentery capillary than in the branch from which it arose, but Whytt argues this is a result of local stimulation.

The secretion of glands is by a similar process of small vessel action.[30] In his essay on nervous diseases, Whytt describes the production of excess pale urine in hysterical women to over-activity of the small vessels of the kidney, and here seems to imply that this organ works partly by blood pressure, speaking of the excretion of bloody urine after exercise and consequent increase of blood pressure in certain pathological cases. He does not make it clear here that he does *not* think of the brain as a gland secreting nervous spirits, though such a belief would not be consistent with his other opinions. Thus, while the kidney may work by blood pressure, 'in other glands, whose structure is finer, particularly the brain and testes . . . .', the motion of fluids is due to oscillation of the small vessels. Before this, he speaks of the 'finest secretory vessels of the brain' in which the fluids cannot move more than one-twelfth of an inch in a second. It is probable that this is a premise for the purposes of argument, as a little later when he says: 'With regard to the nerves, which are generally considered as excretory ducts of the brain; it is probable that the conveyance of their fluid to the various parts of the body is not only owing to a gentle oscillation

[30] They are supplied with bibulous veins, which takes off any improper liquid. Whytt supposed it possible that different veins by the varying nature of their absorbency could take up different fluids, thus providing an explanation of secretion.

in them and their surrounding membranes, but also in some degree to their attraction as capillary tubes; for no sooner can there be a waste of this fluid at the extremity of any nerve (whether this happens from exhalation, alternate compression of the neighbouring parts, or any other cause) than by its attractive power it will be filled again'.[31]

That this is a supposition for purposes of discussion is borne out by Whytt's exposition of the structure of nerves which prefaces the essay on nervous diseases, in which he doubts the existence of any nervous fluid, whether it be to perform the functions of the nerve, or to nourish it.

The return of blood from the fine vessels to the heart, by way of the veins, is aided by the pulsation of neighbouring arteries, the action of the voluntary muscles, and 'the alternate compression made upon all the contents of the abdomen and thorax by the motion of respiration'. Elsewhere when dealing with respiration, Whytt simply adds the pressure in the lungs to the pressure of blood to determine the force of the return of the latter to the heart. The presence of valves in the veins prevents the blood from flowing backward upon the oscillation of the fine vessels.

The ultimate structure of the circulatory system was a matter of some dispute. Borelli for example, as mentioned above, thought the capillaries ended in spongy tissue, and Harvey spoke of 'pores'. Whytt has four possible alternative terminations: the arterial capillaries empty into venous capillaries, serous vessels, the *tela cellulosa* or the cells themselves. Under normal conditions the red corpuscles do not pass through the orifices by which the capillaries communicate to the serous vessels or *tela cellulosa*, but may do so at times of great exertion of the heart.

The emptying of vessels directly into cells is only specifically mentioned in the case of the erection of the penis, a problem occasioning some discussion at the time. Duvernoy and Vieussens had considered that the veins of the organ were constricted by the mechanical action of the nerves, delaying the return of blood (blushing had a similar explanation). Haller and Whytt disagreed. In his essay on vital motions, Whytt explained the matter thus: by the influence of the mind, the blood was propelled with greater force in the small vessels, and ' . . . while such [arteries] as terminate with open orifices in the cells of the penis will through their dilated mouths pour forth not only a serous or lymphatic fluid, as usual, but the red blood itself . . .'[32]

[31] *Works*, p. 238.
[32] Ibid., p. 55.

All such fluids derived from the circulatory system are put forth by exuding arteries and taken up by bibulous veins, particularly in the body cavities, which need lubrication (this from Boerhaave). Such veins deliver to the lymphatics or veins (Monro). It has been noted in hydrocephalus how over-active exhalant arteries produce a dropsy; similarly, lethargic animals become fat as their bibulous veins are insufficiently moved by motion of voluntary muscles to carry away deposits of oils and fats. Such bibulous veins and exhalant arteries are present in the skin and lungs: on average, forty ounces of water are exhaled by these organs in Great Britain and fifty-four in South Carolina (from Dr. Lining). In this way many infectious particles and medicines are taken up. Musschenbroek had shown that air in its gaseous state could not be taken up by the lungs, and Whytt was aware of air in solution, for he speaks of air separating from the blood in morbid states. Apart from his description of 'orifices' too small to be seen, (rather than semi-permeable membranes), admitting fluid but not corpuscles, the lymph functions indeed in this rather 'bibulous' and 'exhalant' way.

Monro junior had demonstrated in fact that lymphatic vessels were absorbent veins, going first to glands. Since absorbent veins in general had no common cavity with arteries, as did other veins, they cannot derive thence a pulse to propel their fluids, and thus Whytt uses them as examples of this theory. Those originating in the gut could be squeezed by its motions, and all fluids would be attracted by the capillary action of these small vessels: Musschenbroek had shown that animal fluids were readily attracted in this way. As other examples of fluids moving in small vessels without aid of the heart, Whytt points to the chick, whose heart, as Malpighi had found, does not beat until the end of the second day, and to the ascent of sap, which is assisted by capillary action and the vibratory motion excited by the heat of the sun, and which is removed at the top of the plant by 'perspiration' at the leaves. Hales had discovered that a vine stem of seven-eighths of an inch in diameter developed a pressure of sap greater by five times than the pressure of blood in the crural artery of a horse. Whytt argues that this is evidence of the power of capillary tubes developed by oscillation: 'And is not the extraordinary force of the sap in the bleeding vine owing to its vessels being susceptible of stronger vibrations than those of most other plants?'.[33]

[33] Ibid., p. 245.

CHAPTER VI

The Controversy with Haller:
Sense and Sensibility.

The major dispute between Whytt and Haller concerned two main issues:

(a) Whytt held that the power of sensibility was widespread in the body, while Haller believed that several organs and tissues were quite insensible. (b) Whytt denied that contractility was an inherent and independent force of the muscular 'glue' as Haller had said, but maintained that the capacity of the muscle to contract depended upon the nerves and the soul.

The debate really began with the publication of Whytt's book on the vital and involuntary motions in 1751. We have seen above (p.9) how Haller criticized the book and Whytt's conception of the central role of the sentient principle, or soul, in physiology. In the same year (1752) as this criticism Haller read two papers to the Royal Society of Sciences of Göttingen on the sensible and irritable parts of the body. This was published as *De Partibus Corporis Humani Sensibilibus et Irritabilibus* in the same year, when there also appeared an inaugural dissertation on the same subject by his pupil Zimmerman.

Haller's paper aroused widespread interest and some opposition, particularly over Haller's claim that the tendons and periosteum were insensible. De Haën energetically opposed this, but 'more important'[1] objections came from Whytt, Le Cat and Delius. The latter two were Stahlians, and it is perhaps in this grouping of his opponents together that we find the origin of Haller's persistent opinion that Whytt was also a Stahlian. Other physicians who repeated Haller's experiments agreed with his results.[2]

No doubt Whytt was stimulated to reply by Haller's unfavourable treatment of his essay on the vital motions both in the book review

---

[1] A. von Haller, *A Dissertation on the Sensibility and Irritability of the Parts of Animals*, London, 1755, reprinted with an introduction by Owsei Temkin, Baltimore, 1936, p. 3.

[2] For example, R. Brocklesby, 'An Account of Some Experiments on the Sensibility and Irritability of the Several Parts of Animals', *Phil. Trans.*, 1755-6, *49*, 240.

and in *De Partibus*. His answer took the form of the second of his *Physiological Essays*, 'Observations of the Sensibility and Irritability of the Parts of Men and other Animals'. This, continues the title page, was 'Occasioned by the celebrated M. de Haller's late Treatise on Those Subjects'.

Haller defended himself against Whytt in *Mémoires sur la Nature sensible et irritable des Parties du Corps animal*, Lausanne, 1756–60, and criticized much of Whytt's work. Whytt added to the second, 1761, edition of his 'Observations . . .', an 'Appendix containing an Answer to M. de Haller', which in the 1768 edition was combined with the essay itself. Haller had the last word in 1764 with a tract *Ad Roberti Whyttii nuperum scriptum Apologia*. Whytt's reputation was such, as Haller admits, that his objections to Haller demanded no small effort to refute them: 'Est autem ea Cl. viri fama, ut non videatur mihi ad ejus objectiones silendum'.[3] Haller did not receive Whytt's *Appendix* until he had published his *Opera Minora* where he would otherwise have defended himself specifically against it. The substance of the dispute in the collected *Works* has less asperity than the previous individual papers, probably due to the editing by Pringle and Whytt's son. Haller's great *Elementa Physiologiae* not only disagrees with Whytt over the action of opium, as we have seen, but also finally rejects Whytt's ideas on irritability.[4]

The argument over sensibility is the more simple of the two. Haller, in *De Partibus* considered the following parts of the body to be insensible: tendons, marrow, aponeuroses, dura and pia mater, ligaments, pleura, capsulae of the articulations, periosteum, peritoneum, bones, pericardium, mediastinum and cornea. This conclusion he reached on experimental evidence, in that animals showed no signs of pain when these parts were stimulated, and that no nerves had been discovered serving these tissues.

In disagreeing with Haller over the sensibility of these organs, Whytt is not entirely dealing in the theoretical side of medicine; he notes that such conclusions are of considerable clinical importance. Whytt has been claimed as the first to notice the inhibitory mechanism of shock in experiments on the nervous system, an observation he had just made in his essay on the vital motions of animals, and which he uses here as an argument against Haller: just as a frog, decapitated, will not move its leg upon stimulation of the foot for some fifteen minutes after decollation, the nervous mechanism of the deeper-lying organs of the body will be inhibited

---

[3] A von Haller, *Ad Roberti Whyttii nuperum scriptum Apologia*, 1764, p. 14.

[4] A. von Haller, *Elementa Physiologiae Corporis Humani*, vol. 4, p. 312 et seq.

by the major operation necessary to reveal them. This will be particularly so in the innermost organs, such as the kidney. Whytt explains this as a greater pain destroying a lesser, and takes his authority from Hippocrates. Nevertheless, an acquaintance of Whytt reported at a nephrotomy that the patient felt pain in his kidneys. Whytt is inclined to attach more importance to such an experiment rather than many more upon animals which are unable to communicate. Stones in the kidney also occasion pain, but not always, as Haller points out.

Whytt claimed great sensibility for the marrow of the bones. Monro junior at an amputation in 1760 had found that the patient, grumbling when the flesh was touched and feeling nothing at the application of a stimulus to the bone, felt great pain when the marrow was touched. Du Verney had experimented with live animals before the Royal Academy of Sciences in Paris at the beginning of the century with similar results, and had had similar experiences to Monro in the hospitals: 'Dans les hôpitaux, oü voyant panser ceux qui avoient eu un bras ou une jambe coupée, je pouvois voir la moille à découvert,—toutes les fois que je la fasiois toucher un peu rudement, le malade donnoit aussitôt de marques d'une nouvelle douleur'.[5]

Haller knew of Du Verney's experiment, but said in *Mémoires sur les Parties sensibles*, vol. 4, p. 109, that a single experiment was insufficient evidence: the marrow was 'cellular' and seemed to have no nerves. Whytt was content to believe that the marrow, being sensible, must have nerves. Haller objected to this type of reasoning: 'It is improper to say that there must be nerves in parts where we cannot see them; the proof of the proposition lies in the observation'.[6]

Haller remained undecided on the sensibility of the marrow, and seems to use something of Whytt's principle of a greater pain destroying a lesser to explain his uncertainty: 'Nam in animale, cui crudelissime oporteat carnes omnes incidere, ut os nudetur, sensum novum doloris aequivorum credo'.[7]

Haller, in his original paper, claimed that all membranes were insensible, including the cornea. Whytt pointed out that the cornea was sensible of a touch of the finger and to tobacco smoke etc. Haller took this up again in the *Mémoires sur les Parties sensibles*, observing that in such a case it is the conjunctiva that is touched, yet

[5] Whytt's *Works*, p. 261.
[6] A. von Haller, *Apologia*, p. 18.
[7] Ibid. In the present volume, generally speaking, all quotations taken from works in Latin have been translated into English unless there is some doubt as to the correct interpretation.

this also is without feeling, the pain being due to a branch of the fifth nerve running between these membranes. Whytt replies, in effect, that nerve endings have to be present for sensibility, and that these membranes are sensible, or at least the conjunctiva. Haller accuses Whytt of inconsistency over this last point, claiming that Whytt had said the cornea was without feeling. Whytt replied with a touch of asperity that he had in fact said this membrane *could* be without feeling, as one may often cut the skin, one of the most sensible organs of the body, while shaving, yet not notice it. Similarly, in operations where the cornea is pierced with a sharp needle, the pain occasioned by holding the eye rigid in the orbit destroys the lesser pain of the incision. Haller cites 'the experiment of Davielus, repeated a thousand times'[8] which shows the cornea to be insensible, and quotes Mekel who dissected branches of the fifth and seventh pair of nerves, between the sclerotic and conjunctiva, up to the edge of the cornea proper: it was likely they remained in the same junction.

Of the arteries, Haller considered only the aorta, temporal, lingual, labial, thyroid and pharyngeal to be sensible. This, as he explains in the *Apologia*, is largely because they have nerves. Whytt, as noted previously, thought all arteries down to capillary size to be sensible. Both agree that sensibility depends upon the presence of nerves. Whytt argues that tendons are in fact muscle and thus have nerves. Haller in the *Mémoires sur les Parties sensibles* claims that Whytt acknowledged sensibility of the tendons simply on this ground, of innervation. Whytt replied that this would be contrary to his assessment of the 'very obtuse feeling' of the tendons.[9] Sensibility, he adds, depends also upon the disposition and state of the nerves; thus the ureters, for example, which they both consider sensible, can be tied without pain, an argument which Haller uses to substantiate his idea of insensible arteries. Such nerves, which in the healthy state, carry a very obtuse or no feeling may become very active in morbid conditions. It this way, argues Whytt, bones, which are normally insensible, but which have nerves, produce when broken a matrix from their substance which is sensible; the dura mater, which Winslow showed to have nerves, and 'which, in a sound state, has but little feeling, granulates after the trepan and feels every irritating substance applied to it, and the same thing happens to cartilages, ligaments, tendons, membranes, etc.'[10] Since

[8] Ibid., p. 17.
[9] Haller lists La Faye, Heister, Garengeot, Boerhaave, Van Swieten and Quesney as thinking the tendons insensible. Bryan Robinson and George Thomson thought otherwise. Crawford, a predecessor of Whytt's, ascribed sympathy to the sensibility of the tendons.
[10] *Works*, p. 267.

he claimed the dura mater to be without feeling, Haller claimed it was not the seat of phrenitis. Whytt describes his own experience and that of Van Swieten of pathological changes in the organ associated with the disease. Brocklesby removed sections of crania from animals and considered both pericranium and dura mater insensible.

Van Swieten described the inflamed tendon of a young nobleman which was so sensitive that it caused convulsions when touched. Brocklesby found the exposed tendo achilles of a sheep to be quite insensible. Haller, writing in the *Apologia* does not seem to have known of Winslow's demonstration of nerves of the dura and pia mater, and denies the existence of such: 'There are certainly no nerves in the hard membrane of the brain . . . No one, I say, with any probable appearance of truth has demonstrated any nerves in this noble membrane, nor in the *pia* membrane, nor in the long integuments of the spinal medulla; Whytt himself offers nothing.'[11]

Whytt develops his idea to cover other parts of the body: inflammation in general is due to the increased oscillation of the small vessels, and this, a muscular motion, presupposes the presence of nerves. The pain of inflammation also derives from the vessels, and is due to nerves. Other examples he gives are joints, which are painful (ligaments and tendons) in rheumatism, contusions on the great trochanter of the thigh, inflammation of the periosteum, suppuration of the marrow, tela cellularis and cornea.

The clinical importance of these theories, as pointed out by Whytt, is exemplified in two operations of the time: bleeding, at the median vein, and a puncture for a dropsy of a joint. The swelling consequent upon the opening of the median vein was due, in Haller's opinion, to damaged nerves, but Whytt, by illustration of cases, shows this is not so, and in other cases is due to the tendo bicipitis. Haller had recommended, in *De Partibus*, a puncture of the capsula in cases of dropsy of the knee. Whytt remarked that this caused a dangerous amount of pain, to which Haller, *Mémoires sur les Parties sensibles*, replied that Mr. Warner advised such a puncture, and that he was a better authority than Whytt. Whytt countered by observing that he had spoken on the authority of Monro senior. Brocklesby had found the capsule of a sheep insensitive to 'pungent liquors and salts', and in general agreed with Haller's results.

Haller, believing membranes insensible, could not accept that the pleura was the seat of pleurisy, and argued that it should be stretched at expiration, whereas the patient felt the most pain at inspiration. Whytt pointed out that not only is the pleura inflamed during pleurisy, but the pleura will in fact be stretched by the

[11] A. von Haller, *Apologia*, p. 16.

diaphragm at inspiration, the intercostal muscles being scarcely used, as Haller himself had shown. Middleton, *ex ipsa America* had moved the back of a scalpel along the uncovered pleura, and found great pain occasioned thereby, but Haller in his *Apologia* claimed this was due to nerves going through the pleura to the muscles of the chest and abdomen.

Haller believed that the skin and subcutaneous nerves played a large part in gout, but Whytt observed that the joints are stiffened and the affected ligaments and tendons are painful. As Haller remarks, Whytt did not mention the experiments of his 'pupil and assistant' Robert Ramsay, 'with Vaughan in the dispute of *Rheumatism*'[12] which seemed to show the tendons insensible. Neither author was aware of, or concerned with, Richard Brocklesby's paper, which was read before the Royal Society in 1756, in which he, by repeating Haller's experiments, concluded that sensibility was very limited in the body. In general, his results agree with those of Haller, although his ideas on irritability and sensibility are less precise than those of Whytt or Haller: 'I laid the pungent liquors and salts, as above upon various parts of the animal, yet alive; as upon the fat, cellular membrane of the neck, leg and other parts within the skin, the liver, pancreas and spleen, and could not find them endowed either with remarkable sensibility or irritability; nor had the bladder any remarkable symptoms of irritability farther than might be occasioned by its muscular fibres'.[13] By these results is he 'induced to coincide with Haller, Castell and Zimmerman, that no part is sensible but the nerves only, and that some parts are irritable without sensibility accompanying them in any degree; whilst others are altogether without sense, whilst at the same time they are incapable of being irritated at all.'[14]

Part of Brocklesby's object was to discover, in future experiments based on this series, whether irritability depended upon a different set of nerves from those which serve voluntary motion and sensation. Such an idea is inherent in that of the reflex and 'sympathy'.

The dispute over irritability was longer. 'Irritability' was the power of a tissue to contract, and Whytt disputed with Haller its nature and origin. Haller claimed that irritability was an inherent property of the 'glue' which with the 'earthy particles' it held together, formed the body of the muscle. To Whytt, this seemed to hover on the edge of an impious and unphilosophical declaration of mechanism:

Some may be of the opinion, that the all-wise Author of nature

[12] Ibid., p. 14.
[13] R. Brocklesby, op cit., p. 240.
[14] Ibid.

hath endued the muscular fibres of animals with certain active powers, far superior to those of common matter, and that to these the motions of irritated muscles are owing. And indeed, we cannot but acknowledge that He has animated all the muscles and fibres of animals with an active SENTIENT PRINCIPLE united to their bodies, and that to the agency of this principle are owing the contractions of stimulated muscles. But if it be imagined that He has given to animal fibres a power of sensation and of generating motion, without superadding or uniting them to an active principle as the SUBJECT and CAUSE of these, we presume to say, that supposition of this kind ought not to be admitted; since to suppose that matter may, of itself, by any modification of its parts, be rendered capable of sensation, or of generating motion, seems to be as unreasonable as to ascribe to it a power of thinking.[15]

In the place of what he considered to be materialistic mechanism Whytt inserted his own physiological doctrine: irritability was a power of the soul which, coextensive with the body, resided in the muscle. Sensibility, just as irritability, could never be the result of an arrangement of matter and so no contraction could result from the advent of a mechanical stimulus upon any mechanical *vis insita*, as Haller had said. Instead, the power of contraction could only be awakened by the sentient activity of the soul in the nerves. The contracting muscle 'perceived' the stimulus, and perception was a property of the sentient principle alone. In this way irritability depended on sensibility, and this upon the nerves. Haller, on the other hand, maintained that irritability was independent of the nerves.

In answer to Whytt's charges of materialism and mechanism, Haller explains that the *vis insita*, although purely mechanical, was no 'mere arrangement of matter' as it derived its powers originally and directly from God. By an ingenious argument he even contrives to appear more pious than Whytt in that he allows no inferior incorporeal forces below God Himself to be responsible for motion: 'I have doubts about this spirit [Whytt's sentient principle] being the cause of motion. I derive all from God'.[16] He also says 'I piously acknowledge that God is the Mover of all nature'.[17] and elsewhere is even more specific: 'Neither the energy of expanding air, nor the weight of a stone, nor the effervescence of acids and alkalis, nor the attractive power of a dissected muscle can be referred to incorporeal

---

[15] *Works*, p. 128.
[16] A. von Haller, *Apologia*, p. 27.
[17] A. von Haller, *Elementa Physiologiae Corporis Humani*, vol. 4, p. 183.

forces. God gave to bodies this attractive power and other forces, which once accepted are exercised; nor are they owing to any soul or spirit below God.'[18]

Whytt, of course, *did* allow inferior immaterial agencies; not only the soul of man, but also incorporeal 'intelligencies' in some way responsible for that soul. Haller was almost in the position of Descartes and Locke, who had said that it was in God's power to give sentience to matter if He so wished. And having done so, added Haller, He had no need to be further concerned in the maintenance of sense or motion, which was now simple mechanism. Whytt, conversely, needed the perpetual activity of an incorporeal force to explain physiological phenomena.

In answer to a criticism of Whytt's, Haller explains that the muscular glue contains, of itself, the origins or rudiments of the *vis insita*, by which he seems to mean the necessary arrangements, the material cause, as it were: 'The rudiments of the contractile nature are in the gluten: step by step animal motion rises from the contractile nature to the *vis insita* and from that to the nervous force.'[19]

Thus the whole dispute over irritability centred around the *nature* of irritability—whether it was a characteristic of matter, or of a life-force—and its relationship to sensibility. Haller, of course, recognized that in the usual processes of physiology muscular contraction was generally brought about by the advent of a disturbance in the nerves, from 'voluntary' or 'involuntary' sources, but he nevertheless maintained that contractility and sensibility were distinct phenomena which could occur without reference to each other. This strict denial of any relationship between sensibility and irritability left him unable to make use of the elaborations of it which Whytt[20] successfully employed in considering the idea of the reflex and sympathy.

Haller gives examples of those cases where he considered that irritability was independent.

But I remove several motions of muscles from the nervous force. For who can refer to the nerves the retractive force seen under the knife in a muscle excised from the body three days ago, and now semi-putrid? Who can restore to the soul the irritable force of intestines cut from the body, when those intestines are remote

---

[18] Ibid.

[19] A. von Haller, *Apologia*, p. 25.

[20] As Temkin observes (in the introduction to the Baltimore, 1936, reprint of the English version of Haller's paper on sensibility and irritability) that Whytt was correct in opposing the radical distinction of irritability and sensibility, which left no room for concepts such as the reflex.

70

from the *imperium* of the soul? Who, lastly, can attribute to the nerves that *vis insita* which is so eminently displayed in the living animal whether the nerves are ligatured or removed?[21]

Sed vermibus, sed classi testaceae, sed mentulis, hydris, aliisque Zoophytis, millies eruca majoribus, nulli sunt nervi . . . In grandi Animali, viribus insignibus, ut in polypo maris mediterrano per A. KOELREUTERUM . . . dissecto, nullum cerebrum, nullos nervos inventos esse, id ad demonstrationem irritabilis natura esse absque nervo.[22]

In the first of these we have a clue to the centre of the whole dispute. As Haller said later, when summing up a discussion on the seat of the soul, the controversy rests on the definition of sensation. Throughout these publications Haller reserves the adjective 'sensible' for those organs or tissues which are capable of communicating to the soul within the brain and there arousing a conscious sensation. He therefore never accepted Whytt's notion of *unconscious* sensation, a mere lowly animal 'feeling' of the sort that allowed oysters to close up at the approach of danger. This unconscious sensation existed within a stimulated nerve only; muscular contraction could not occur without its previous activity; and in decapitated animals it was sufficient to produce complex motions from an organizing centre such a the spinal cord. In *all* cases it was a faculty of that part of the coextensive soul which inhabited the nerves, and for this reason it was a psychic faculty. This is what Haller objected to (as we may see in the above quotation) because he insisted the soul was in the brain only, and that the *vis insita* would account for the other appearances. His principal objection concerned the more extreme case of the isolated muscle, which he said was moved by a stimulus and the *vis insita* and which Whytt said both felt and moved by what at first sight appeared to be a divided soul. Whytt felt himself to be most open to attack on the subject of the divisibility of the soul, and argued (not very convincingly) that his doctrine did not make this assumption. Haller was more than ever convinced that movements of isolated members were evidence only of a purely material mechanism: 'That an amputated arm or an excised intestine can reach my soul and be animated by it is so remote from all probability that even my opponents must reject this part of the Whyttian doctrine'.[23]

Thus all of those processes, from simple stimulation of an excised muscle to the retraction, mediated by the spinal cord, of the

[21] A. von Haller, *Apologia*, p. 19.
[22] [23] Ibid., p. 20.

stimulated toe of a headless frog, which Whytt attributed to unconscious perception and subsequent action on the part of the sentient principle, were for Haller the complex result of material activity, and none of them entered into his definition of sentient activity, which in most cases we can equate with sensibility. As their definitions of the subject did not coincide to some extent they were talking at cross-purposes, at least in the theoretical counterpart to their observations.

On the more practical side of the discussion however the difficulties were not so pronounced: the method of discovering whether a part was sensible was to stimulate it with a scalpel or acid. If the animal responded with obvious struggles, then, they would have agreed, the part was sensible. On this basis Haller made three observations on which depended his axiom that irritability is independent of sensibility. These were:

    (a) The most sensitive parts of the body, nerves and skin, are not irritable.

    (b) Irritability is not proportional to sensibility.

    (c) Some parts are irritable but have no feeling.

The first of these shows that Haller is arguing on a much wider basis than Whytt, and when he uses it to reject Whytt's idea that irritability *is* proportional to sensibility, Whytt is able to show that his proposition referred to more limited and precise circumstances than Haller had imagined: the irritable parts of the skin are naturally enough the muscles present in it, and in their reactions to stimuli—in raising goose-pimples and inflammations—irritability could be shown to be proportional to sensibility. In more general terms, Whytt had envisaged the sensibility of the nerve, in the simplest situation, to be proportional to the irritability of the muscle, so that Haller's remark that nerves were not irritable was no valid objection. It betrays, indeed, a misunderstanding of Whytt's carefully thought out physiological scheme. Again, Haller argues that the stomach is more sensitive than the intestines, but less irritable. Whytt once more insists that contractility is a property only of muscle and sensitivity only of nerves, and considerations involving the balance between the two forces should most properly be limited to the two tissues. Haller, taking organs rather than tissues as the basis of his argument, was on dangerous ground, but could not limit himself as Whytt had done, for he imagined that sensibility was not a unique property of nerves, as it could exist without them (but was therefore difficult to assign with any confidence to any other type of tissue); and that the difficulty of relating such an uncertain quality to irritability was reduced to an impossibility by the fact that certain animals could be shown to have no nerves at all, as in the case of Koelreuter's polyp (p.71).

The third of these points of Haller's show very clearly what he meant by sensibility. The parts which are irritable but have no (or very little) feeling are principally the muscles of which the most important was the heart. Haller did not doubt of course that an exposed muscle would be stimulated into action by a stimulus, but this was mechanism; the real test was to discover whether *sensation* followed such a stimulus. This was not entirely a rhetorical question, for both authors recalled that Harvey had touched the living heart of a 'nobleman' and found it insensible. Whytt suggested that Harvey had actually handled the insensible *callus* surrounding the heart, but Haller added the anecdote to his list of personal experiments in which he found that stimulation of the exposed hearts of a variety of animals caused no indications of great pain. The heart was thus not very sensible, but clearly very irritable. How, asked Haller, is that to be explained? In the first place, answered Whytt, the outside of the heart, *callus* or not, is clearly not meant to be so sensible as the inside, where the returning blood stimulates it into renewed motion, where a feverish humour may cause a desperate pulse, and where, in the excised heart of an animal, it may be so sensitive that a warm breath may renew its action.

Whytt brought two other arguments to bear against Haller's doctrine of the independence of irritability. The first of these concerned the action of opium. Whytt held that opium acted directly upon the nerves, having an inhibitory effect. He came to this conclusion from observations on the rapidity of its action and experiments mentioned in the account of his paper on opium given in chapter 5 (p.50), where also are described Haller's objections.

The outcome was Whytt's conclusion that opium rendered an animal languid or paralytic purely by lessening sensitivity. Opium, he said, when injected into the stomach of an experimental animal, caused paralysis of the muscles *before* it could reach them, by its direct action on the nerves on which irritability so absolutely depended. If irritability were independent, why should not a muscle remain irritable upon a direct stimulus before the opium which was already acting upon the nerves had yet reached it?

The second argument suggested that if irritability were a property of the muscular glue, then contraction at a direct stimulus to the muscle would be greater than to a stimulus relayed sympathetically by the nerves. Pricking the toe of a frog with a needle brings about a greater contraction of the muscle concerned in withdrawing the foot than if that muscle itself were stimulated directly. Surely this would not be the property of a mechanical force?

Whytt allied this second argument to a more powerful third. We have already seen how he employed the dictum 'a greater pain destroys a lesser' to explain why the operation to expose organs obscured their sensibility, and here he applies it to irritability. The great pain occasioned by cutting off the head of a frog destroys for a while all lesser pains: the animal is insensible and consequently immobile. Direct or sympathetic stimulation of a muscle does not produce a contraction. If the muscular glue were purely mechanical and non-sensible, then there could be no question of its sensibility being destroyed in this way and its contraction would proceed as usual.

Haller does not seem to have an answer to this, the phenomenon of shock probably being new to him. To acquaint himself with the experimental observations which Whytt used as a basis for argument, he wrote to Caldani asking him to decapitate a frog and observe the results of experiments on it. Caldani wrote back[24] to say that he could not generate convulsions by pressing the exposed section of the spinal cord until three or four minutes had passed, and that stimuli applied to the hind leg produced no result before half an hour had elapsed. These results coincide with Whytt's, and it is not clear what use Haller made of them.

The remainder of the dispute is taken up with a consideration of what organs are irritable, and rests on purely practical observations. Haller allowed irritability to lacteal veins, mucus glands and sinuses and denied it to arteries, veins, and excretory ducts.

Whytt, defending the ideas of the first of these two *Physiological Essays*, argued that the small vessels showed their irritability in blushing, inflammation etc. Haller countered this in his *Mémoires sur les Parties sensibles* by claiming such activity would result in these vessels emptying themselves. In the *Apologia* he rests his case by saying that no appearance of irritability or sensibility is seen if a small vessel is cleanly cut with a sharp scalpel.

Haller was likewise unable to find any irritability of the aorta or vena cava by pricking them. Whytt replied that while the muscle coat appeared tendinous, yet the mucus glands and sinuses, which Haller allowed to be irritable, had the same appearance. The apparent pulsations of the vena cava, claimed Haller, were due to blood pushed back into it from the auricle. Whytt cited Steno, who saw the vena cava in a rabbit contract some six or seven times before the auricle. Haller seems ultimately to have been convinced of this.

Whytt argued for the irritability of the kidney by claiming that its

---

[24] L. M. A. Caldani, *Ad Hallerum Epistola*, Venice, 1764, p. 7.

sudden production of great quantities of pale urine in hysteric cases was due to the increased activity of its small vessels. Haller had thought other glands, the lachrymal, and mucus sinuses were irritable on a similar basis, that they increased production upon stimulation, yet he denied irritability to the kidney.

The excretory ducts were more open to experiment: Haller poured oil of vitriol on to a ureter and observed no movement, while Whytt stated that a stone in this part causes contraction. (Monro junior saw a ureter contract in a half-dead pig.) Haller makes a comparison with the pupil, which does not contract when touched, yet is clearly mobile. Haller explains this by denying muscular power to the uvea, as the pupil widens after death. It has no orbicular muscle and its motion is due to the inflow of fluid. Whytt, of course, insisted that as it moved it must have a muscle. Although Haller uses it as an example of irritability without sensibility, Whytt was able to show with such precision that the sensibility of the *retina* was absolutely necessary for this motion and proportional to it, that it became known as Whytt's reflex.

Although Whytt's experiments and theoretical explanations of 'simple sensation' depending on local nerves and, in other cases, the spinal marrow, were instrumental in developing the reflex theory, it is interesting to see that Whytt uses the expression 'reflex act' to mean almost exactly the opposite to the involuntary unconscious act of modern physiology: '[Simple sensation] will not be attended with what is called consciousness . . . because this reflex act, by which a person knows his thoughts or sensations to be his own, is a faculty of the soul exercised in the brain only'.[25]

Pursuant to this and by way of summary, we may anticipate a little the subject of a later chapter and mention that the sentient principle which Whytt imagined to be at the centre of these actions was bound to the body by several 'laws of union' by which in all but voluntary actions it was compelled to act in predetermined ways. This central conception gives him a flexible physiological scheme which combines rigid laws with an idea of the organic unity of the animal, tending towards its preservation.

Thus Whytt finds a relationship between irritability and sensibility which is fixed but elaborate enough to produce such fruitful conceptions as the reflex and 'sympathy'. In a sense his whole physiology stands upon this relationship and its elaborations, the most important of which is the statement that sensibility and irritability may be spatially distinct. Other details are arrived at step by step: sensibility may occur alone; irritability is always preceded

[25] *Works*, p. 287.

by sensibility; sensibility is the unique property of nerves, irritability of muscles; if the site of sensibility is identical with that of irritability, the latter is simple and fixed; and if the site of sensibility is distant then a sympathetic organizing centre (the spinal cord or brain) intervenes and the resultant action is complex.

The whole of Whytt's system of voluntary and involuntary motions is fully discussed in the next chapter, and the present one may be concluded by a list of points of interest for contemporary physiologists compiled by Haller in summarizing Whytt's side of the argument. This may be compared to the list given above which may, at the discretion of the critical reader of Whytt's works, be considered to be of interest to the modern historian.

1. The greater pain of operating upon an animal obscures the sensibility of the tendons;

2. Tendons and the dura mater have obtuse feeling in health, but are more sensible when inflamed, and that the dura mater has nerves;

3. Irritability cannot exist without sensibility;

4. The soul feels, unconsciously, over all the body;

5. The soul exists in detached members;

6. All animals possess nerves, and a head or something analogous;

7. A decapitated frog moves, and withdraws its foot upon stimulation. *ex consilio;*

8. Irritation (*irritatio*) causes inflammation rather than blockage;

9. Opium slows the heart;

10. The vena cava is not irritable.

CHAPTER VII

Involuntary Motions and the Reflex

In making a study of the involuntary motions of animals Whytt made some observations which were important in the development of the idea of reflex action. This study, *An Essay on the Vital and Other Involuntary Motions of Animals*, Edinburgh, 1751, must be regarded as Whytt's most important work. It sets out the doctrine of his physiology, which in his other works, has been described in previous chapters; and the peculiar importance of the soul, which is dealt with more thoroughly in later chapters. Whytt described three types of animal motion: (i) voluntary; (ii) involuntary; (iii) mixed.

Voluntary motions proceeded from an activity of the will, involuntary were those over which the will had no influence, such as the contraction of the pupil and the beating of the heart (which was specifically one of a number of 'vital' motions), and the term 'mixed' covered those motions, like respiration, which could be temporarily modified, but not permanently governed by the will.

Unlike most of his contemporaries, Whytt did not search for a mechanical explanation of muscle contraction, but attributed it to the 'sentient principle' or soul, which, distributed all over the body, was empowered to initiate motion only in the muscles. In all cases, this sentient principle was made to act by a stimulus arriving at the muscle. This process required the sensitive action of the soul, a capacity of it exercised only in the nerves, the agents of feeling.

This stimulus could arise naturally or experimentally at the muscle, or could be the usual nerve impulse. In experimental cases, the stimulus could be a physical or chemical disturbance. Even in the case of a muscle stimulated into contraction by pricking it with a pin, Whytt seems to have envisaged sufficient nervous material existing within the body of the muscle to account for its sensitivity. The contraction resulting from such a stimulus was absolutely involuntary, even in the case of a voluntary muscle. This is principally how Whytt supposed the soul to act in a necessary and obligatory way.

He noticed several particulars regarding the stimulation of exposed muscle which indicate his interest in the problem of how the soul worked, even in isolated muscles. He saw that on a direct stimulus, applied continuously, an exposed muscle did not contract continuously, but alternately relaxed and contracted. This would probably now be attributed to its refractory period. He also noticed that a muscle may remain contracted for a brief space after the cause of stimulation has been removed, and that the stretching of the muscle may act as a stimulus to further contraction. In the case, however, of the stimulus arriving at the muscles naturally, by way of the nerves, (which process, with the exception of that in the voluntary nerves, Whytt speaks of frequently as 'sympathy') the resulting contraction could be continuous. The cause of this phenomenon lay in the fixed way the sentient principle was joined to the body: in the case of a stimulus arriving directly at the muscle, the resulting alternate motions of the muscle would be the most advantageous to throw off the offending cause, whereas the stimulus arriving via the nerves was less likely to have its origin in such a situation, but would rather be a normal physiological mechanism. The cause, if offending, might be for example, the stimulus of the faeces acting sympathetically upon the muscles of the diaphragm to produce a steady contraction, best designed to remove the begetter of the stimulus.

This, then, is the mechanism of all of the involuntary motions described by Whytt. In this way, all muscular contraction could be said to be one of three types: firstly natural contraction, exhibited by certain muscles without antagonists, such as sphincters, where the usual state was contraction rather than relaxation, secondly voluntary, and thirdly, by advent of stimuli. It is with the third type that Whytt was principally involved. The motion of the heart was caused by the stimulating nature of the blood exciting the heart to expel it; the lungs were thrown into activity by the unpleasant stimulus of the air remaining too long in them; food provoked the peristaltic and defecatory motions of the gut; the eye and ear accommodated themselves to excess of light or sound, and the movements of the egg in the oviduct and the semen at coition were owing to their stimulation of the organs containing them.

In this way Whytt reduced all involuntary motions to a simple sequence of events: the stimulating object or circumstance exciting the sentient principle into initiating motion designed (by the Creator rather than the soul) to remove that object or circumstance. The impulses or stimuli entering and leaving the sentient principle were carried by nerves. Since the soul acted in an obligatory, predetermined way, the operation was as automatic as a mechanical explanation, and may be described as quasi-mechanism. In pursuing this idea, Whytt suggested that the magnitude of the stimulus entering the sentient principle was reflected in the extent of the resultant action. The soul resident in the muscles was not, however, the sole arbiter determining the nature and extent of the motion: the soul in its sensitive capacity in the nerves exercised a similarly pre-established discretion as to the kind of stimulus it admitted to influence the soul in its executive capacity. In this way, the same stimulus (that, for example, afforded by cold water) would have very different effects upon different organs (the stomach, in this example, and the lungs).

All the involuntary motions described by Whytt were, then, of two kinds: either the stimulus arrived directly at the muscle, as in the case of the heart, or sympathetically by way of the spinal cord. The importance of this will be seen when the reflex is considered in greater detail.

It was Whytt's early dissatisfaction (from about 1739) with the current theories of the mechanism of respiration and the action of the heart that first turned his ideas to physiology and the functioning of the soul, and we may suppose that the conclusions he came to provided him with one of the two foundations of his entire doctrine of the soul, the other being the observation of the continued life of severed parts of the body.

It is thus of interest to look a little more closely at Whytt's interpretation of these two fundamental physiological activities.

He did not believe that air contained a *pabulum vitae* which was absorbed into the blood at respiration. He differed in this from several of his contemporaries, who probably derived their opinion from Newton and Boyle. He was aware that animals in an enclosed space suffocated, but attributed it to the accumulation of noxious gases, which resembled those of subterranean cavities. The function of respiration was to cool the blood and aid in circulation: 'During inspiration and expiration, the blood finds an easy passage through the vessels of the lungs, as by their alternate inflation and contraction, it is pressed forward to the left ventricle of the heart. After inspiration is completed, it begins to flow with more difficulty; and at the end of expiration, its motion is still less free.'[1]

The blood thus remaining in the vessels of the lungs occasioned an unpleasant sensation which acted upon the sentient principle to renew the inspiration. This could be suppressed for a brief period of time by an effort of will; hence the mixed character of the motion. Anything which lessened the sensibility of the *sensorium* or nerves (such as disease, or a drug like opium) would have a similar effect of suppressing the beginning of inspiration. He described pathological

[1] *Works*, p. 94.

79

conditions where as much as half a minute could elapse between the end of expiration and the beginning of inspiration. The part which the will (that is, the conscious part of the soul) played in respiration, enabling inspiration or expiration to be temporarily suspended, convinced him that the entire process was controlled by the unconscious activity of the same soul. In this way he opposed Boerhaave, who had supposed the expansion of the lungs compressed and rendered inoperative the nerves reaching the thorax, and that the resultant loss of muscular power was the cause of expiration.

Whytt was at some pains to contradict Brémond, who in 1739 drew the conclusion from a series of experiments, that the lungs were capable of inflating themselves under their own power. Whytt (*Works*, p. 82) gives the reference as '*Mémoires de l'Académie des Sciences*, 1739.' Brémond perforated the thorax of several dogs and attempted to observe the lungs directly. Hérissant, five years later, concluded that the lungs were erected by pressure of blood, independently of the thorax. Whytt insisted that only muscles were capable of motion, and that the structure of the lungs did not allow for the kind of observation which Brémond seems to have made. Possibly, argued Whytt, the air contained in the lungs while the dog attempted to cry out would cause them for a short while to emerge from the hole in the thorax, and give the appearance of acting independently of the thorax.

Just as Whytt's sentient principle provided an explanation of the restarting of the heart after stoppage, which was not available to the mechanists, so did it suggest a means whereby another phenomenon could be accounted for. This was the problem of how the newly-born infant began to breathe. This was particularly difficult to explain upon mechanical principles, like those of Boerhaave, and it had long been an opportunity for the animists to demonstrate the wise workings of the soul, which idea seems to go back to the Stoic *pneuma* adherents, who held that the soul was contained in the air, and was drawn into the blood at respiration. At all events, it was only with this first act of the infant that the soul demonstrated its presence, and could be regarded, as if not absent before it, then latent.

Whytt was equally impressed by the inability of matter to initiate motion, which seemed to him to be the strongest possible argument that the motions of respiration were owing to the soul. Nevertheless, there were anatomical questions to be settled: how was it that the infant did not first drown in the amniotic liquor, and second asphyxiate in the air after birth, if prevented from breathing? This was a problem which perplexed Harvey, according to Whytt, who was able to show that at birth the *ductus arteriosus* and the *foramen ovale* closed, and that the blood, having before birth undergone the 'action of the air'[2] by proxy, as it were, in the lungs of the mother, was now forced into pulmonary arteries and lungs. The ultimate and timely cause of the infant's first breath was the manifest appetite of the sentient principle for air.

Boerhaave had postulated for the heart a mechanism similar to that accounting for the motions of the lungs. Whytt succinctly explains it:

> The theory of the heart's motion which has of late years met with the most favourable impression is that of the celebrated Boerhaave, who deduces the alternate systole and diastole of this muscle chiefly from the peculiar circumstance of the cardiac nerves, for as much of the greatest part of these nerves passes between the auricles and the large arteries of the heart, he concluded that they must be compressed at the end of every systole . . . whence the motion of the spirit being intercepted, the heart must be rendered paralytic; but whenever . . . this compression ceases, and the nerves transmit their fluid as formerly, the heart must contract anew.[3]

Morgnani had objected that other nerves passing close to major arteries do not produce alternate motions; a criticism Whytt accepted and to which he added five more: all cardiac nerves do not pass between the auricles and the large arteries; the pressure required to paralyse a nerve is considerable, as in the case of the ulnar nerve, and probably greater than that produced by the heart; the compression of such a nerve as the ulnar does not have immediate effect; such a hypothetical squeezing of the supposedly hollow nerve would inject greater quantities of fluid, momentarily, into the heart, and finally, the single ventricle of fishes contracts regularly and after its abstraction from the body, upon ceasing motion, as in higher animals, the ventricle (left in higher animals) stops first. Whytt had objected to a similar theory of De Gorter that it was difficult to see how the heart could be speeded up on such a mechanism.[4] The system of spirits had its weakest point in the production of energy. It was quite clear, as Whytt had shown elsewhere, that the energy produced by a muscle was far in excess of that which could be given to it by the influx of spirits. Stephen Hales had shown that the blood lost nine-tenths of its 'momentum' at every circulation, and Whytt argued that the heart, and lungs to a lesser extent, must therefore be a source of energy. This could not

[2] Ibid., p. 111.

[3] *An Essay on the Vital and other Involuntary Motions of Animals*, p. 27.

[4] Borelli had also postulated a mechanical heart, involving the discharge of the nervous fluid at nerve endings one drop at a time.

81

be purely 'mechanical', first, because it was not a property of matter to generate energy, and second, on the Cartesian system the blood driven from the heart returned to it in the form of spiritis to provide its motion; this would be perpetual motion, an impossible situation. Similarly the revival of motion in the heart of hibernators cannot be mechanical, but must be due to a sentient principle.

The theory which Whytt put in place of this was his typical quasi-mechanical chain of cause and effect, by which all the vital motions of animals were occasioned. Firstly, the blood returning to the heart acted as a stimulus to that organ, by way of its nerves. In other vital actions, this stimulus was usually described by Whytt as 'unpleasant' to the organ concerned, with the result that the organ was moved into activity designed to rid it of the unpleasant stimulus.

That the returning blood might act as a stimulus to the heart was not a new idea, and Whytt quoted two paragraphs, from Harvey and Glisson, to illustrate this. Haller was also aware of it, and while Sénac ascribed the stimulating nature of blood to its momentum, weight and distending effect, Whytt adds to these causes the chemical nature and heat of the blood. Thus the blood consists of fixed and semivolatile salts (both of which were known to irritate nervous parts), neutral vegetable oils and acrid aromatic oils, and alcohol, 'ardent spirits'. Heat, which 'seems to be no more than a quick vibration or motion in the smaller parts of bodies' increases the stimulating properties of these constituents.

These stimuli acted upon the nerves of the heart. As, however, the blood does not act similarly upon the nerves of other organs, Whytt suggested the qualitative difference lay in the nature of different nerves: 'The nerves of different organs in the same animal are so constituted as to be very differently affected even by the same things'.[5] This is the first appearance of the ideas which anticipated the theory of the specific energy of nerves. The difference had to be within the nerves. The stimulus of the blood was constant in different organs, and the sentient principle acting as a necessary agent had to act if stimulated. The difference lay between the two.

This is the major point of Whytt's theory. He replaced the mechanism of matter with a quasi-mechanical animism. The immaterial principle intermediate between the incoming disturbance of the nerves and the consequent outgoing, executive disturbance, determining the direction and amount of that latter

[5] *Works*, p. 28.

impulse, yet according to pre-determined 'laws' was a new idea, and compromised between the old mechanical theories and the older animist ideas.

To summarize, then, Whytt explained all involuntary motions either by the direct action of the stimulus upon the motor organ, or its indirect action, sympathetically effected by the intervention of the spinal cord, the seat of all sympathy. Although such actions as the withdrawal of the leg of a decapitated frog upon stimulation was sympathetic, Whytt, with the physiology of the time, limited the phrase 'sympathetic organ' and frequently the term 'sympathy' itself, to the viscera. This is a recognition of the difference between what is usually meant by 'reflex', i.e. of the external organs and the action of the sympathetic system: internal reflexes. Whytt's explanation of motions caused by the direct advent of a stimulus may be justified in some cases, notably his description of the mechanism of peripheral circulation (but not, for example that of the motion of the heart), by the modern account of 'axon reflexes', that is to say, those whose nervous connections do not reach the spinal cord. Whytt also accurately described habits, and those motions that became involuntary through habitual usage. Franklin Fearing[6] describes Whytt's account of salivation at the sight of 'grateful food' as an anticipation of the conditioned reflex.

Whytt is best known for his contribution to the development of the idea of the reflex, for reasons which, perhaps, have been wrongly emphasized. They will be discussed, with a brief introduction to the earlier development of the idea, in this section.

For our purposes the history of the reflex begins with Descartes. He first and most completely separated involuntary motions from the soul, which he located in the pineal gland[7] but he described pathways of spirits in involuntary action which did not approach this. The same nerves were sensory and motor. The external object, impinging on the sense organ, pulled a thread within the nerve. This opened the orifices to several other similar nerves, located on the surface of the ventricles, and animal spirit was allowed to flow down them. The principal recipient of the spirits was the nerve going to the organ concerned, in order to remove that organ from danger, but accessory nerves applied the hand to the part and turned the head to observe the cause.

The structure was hypothetical, possibly out of deference to church authorities, possibly because Descartes was a philosopher rather than a physiologist. It was attended with great difficulties in detail,

[6] F. Fearing, op. cit., pp. 80, 282.
[7] Good illustrations of this are found in R. Descartes, *De Homine*, Leyden, 1662, pp. 78, 79.

but owed its influence to its comprehensive nature, providing in one scheme an answer to many problems of physiology.

One such detail concerned muscle contraction. Descartes supposed the animal spirits to be very fine and subtle, and that they flowed down the nerve, between its wall and the enclosed thread, and inflated the muscle like a balloon. The volume of spirits required for a large muscle would be considerable and the rapidity of its contraction made the motion of such a fluid along a nerve of microscopic dimension in such a short time scarcely credible. Willis invented a theory to obviate this difficulty by imagining that the spirits of the nerves were qualitatively different from those of the muscles, and an explosion occurred upon the meeting of the two. Swammerdam clearly showed that a muscle does not increase in volume on contraction, but seems to have been ignored by his contemporaries. Descartes himself, elsewhere, owned that spirits by entering, 'or even only as they tend to enter more or less unto this or that nerve have the power of changing the form of the muscle'.[8]

One of Descartes' examples of the mechanical action and arrangement of the nerves was the behaviour of the pupil in accommodating to near and far sight. That is, by conscious volition, the pineal moved in such a way as to determine spirits into nerves associated with altering the position and accommodation of the eye— dilatation of the pupil—only when that volition concerned the desire to observe distant objects. By no conscious means was it possible to directly dilate the pupil: there was no nervous pathway.

Whytt was also concerned with the dilatation of the pupil in darkness, and the action (Whytt's reflex) was as mechanical as Descartes'. He insisted that the retina was the sensitive part of the eye: an increase in light intensity brought about an unpleasant 'sensation' in the retina, just as air too long in the lungs or blood in the heart, and this was communicated to the sentient principle which at once initiated those motions proper to lessen the offending cause, that is, the pupil narrowed. Anatomy insisted that this action had to be referred to the brain:

> Since the optic nerves and those of the uvea arise from different parts of the brain, and have no communication with each other on their course to the eye, it seems evident that light affecting the retina cannot excite the sphincter into contraction by any immediate mechanical change which it produces either in the muscle itself or in the nerves which actuate it; but the uneasy sensation occasioned in the retina by the admission of too much

[8] From Fearing, op. cit., p. 20.

84

light into the eye, may so affect the sentient principle, which is present and ready wherever the nerves have their origin, as to excite it to contract the orbicular muscle of the area in order to lessen the pupil and exclude the offending cause.[9]

As in all Whytt's involuntary actions, the sentient principle acted as a necessary agent, according to rules of the union of body and soul, not as a conscious principle. This action has all the marks of a reflex: it is rapid, automatic, defensive and unlearned. Whytt believed, like Descartes, that a voluntary effort to see more clearly at close distances narrowed the pupil, but that this could not be achieved by direct volition.

The natural position of the iris was open, to which state it returned by elasticity in rest or darkness. (Not by pressure of the aqueous humour, as Haller said, as this would be equal on both sides of the uvea.) There was great sympathy between the eyes: if one pupil, covered, enlarged in darkness so would the other in a constant intensity of light. Whytt reinforced his argument by relating a case of hydrocephalus, where, the retina being rendered insensible by pressure on the head of the optic nerve, the pupils remained immobile in a dilated state.

After Descartes in the seventeenth century the history of the reflex falls into two main stages. The first describes its treatment at the hands of men who considered the soul to have two distinct 'layers' of action—conscious and unconscious, in the latter of which fall involuntary motions. This group is overshadowed by Descartes and only served to modify his mechanism with a degree of animism.

The second stage involved localization of function: the giving of a locality to the unconscious sensation and motion.

Descartes had indeed located his conscious perception at the pineal and unconscious perception with accompanying motion within the ventricles, i.e. the point of reflection. Willis' point of reflection, as is noted below, was his *sensorium commune*, the *corpora striata*. Only if reflection took place above this, in the *corpus callosum*, was conscious perception involved. However, the involuntary motions originated from the cerebellum and reflected actions could take place there equally as in the cerebrum.

The observations of Boyle that insects could live and procreate after loss of their heads; of Perrault that a dog survived the loss of its brain (also Vieussens and Bohn); of Duverney and Chirac on acephalous monsters; to say nothing of similar observations from Asclepiades to Leonardo (who having removed all the vital

[9] *Works*, p. 64.

85

organs of a frog, considered the spinal cord to be the foundation of life)[10] all fostered a belief, as noted above, that the brain was not the sole organ of sense and motion, and that the medulla spinalis and cerebellum were probably more important to the more essential motions than the cerebrum. Important among such physicians was Preston, who had experience of monsters[11] and experiments involving the removal of the brain from dogs, which nevertheless survived; vitiation of the medulla spinalis caused sudden death. Bohn also experimented with decapitated frogs. It will be seen below that when Whytt argues for a soul extended to the spinal cord, he makes a list of experiments and observations, his own as well as those from Kaau, Boyle, Bacon, Redi, Caldesi, Ridley and Baglivi, all of whom emphasize the importance of this organ.

Thus Whytt's attention was drawn to the spinal medulla. Much of his writings emphasize its importance, and his interest was increased by a communication from his friend and correspondent, Stephen Hales: 'The late Reverend and learned Dr. Hales informed me that having many years since, tied a ligature about the neck of a frog to prevent any effusion of blood, he cut off its head, and thirty hours after, observed the blood circulating freely in the web of the foot; the frog also at this time moved its body when stimulated: but that on thrusting a needle down the spinal marrow, the animal was strongly convulsed and immediately after became motionless.'[12]

The 'fundamental'[13] experiment of finding that the feet of a decapitated frog were still irritable was thus performed by Hales and published by Whytt; Stuart had been the first to confirm it. Whytt's contributions were to show that *only a segment* of the cord was necessary, that inhibition due to shock persisted in the cord for a while after decollation, and to describe *tonus*.[14]

Whytt clearly was fully convinced of the importance of the nerve cord, and was aware of the observations of Duverny and Chirac. He was inclined to grant it a degree of autonomy: it derived its powers not only from the brain but from the particular secretion of its own vessels. Connection of nerves and to a lesser extent of the

[10] K. D. Keele, *Anatomies of Pain*, Oxford, 1957, p. 60.
[11] C. Preston, 'Account of a child born without a brain', *Phil. Trans.*, 1695-7, *19*, 215-35.
[12] *Works*, p. 290.
[13] C. Singer, and E. A. Underwood, *A Short History of Medicine*, Oxford, 1962, p. 251.
[14] Fearing, op. cit., p. 48, observes that Whytt's description of tonus was 'significant'. A similar idea, however, seems to have been common property among many animists, particularly Stahlians, for example Gohl. Whytt's differed in being attributed solely to nervous activity.

spinal medulla with the brain was, in local motion, needed only to keep them fit to be acted on by impulses. He recognized from experiments of Langrish and Schwenke that should the spinal marrow be starved of blood, then paralysis of the lower legs would follow. He was impressed with the comparative anatomy of the question: animals with diffuse nervous systems withstood the loss of the head best, as with Boyle's insects; and among vertebrates those least affected were those with large spinal marrows, like Redi's tortoises, which lived six months; then cats and dogs, which survived several hours, and lastly man, where the influence of the spinal cord enabled the heart, in the absence of the brain, to perform only a few beats. ('Where the soul seems chiefly to act upon the different parts by means of their connection to the brain and spinal marrow'.)[15]

Whytt's idea was derived from the theory of nervous spirits. He does indeed specifically reject that theory, by saying that should he ever use the term 'nervous spirit' then it was to be taken only as 'influence or power of the nerves', but in a few cases the construction of his words seem to imply that the spinal medulla was a reserve of spirits, to some extent capable of generating its own. On the whole, however, it is clear that on such occasions Whytt has merely slipped into an older method of expressing himself.

Both the idea that only a section of the spinal cord is necessary and that it is a reserve of nervous power were expressed by Mayow in 1670, a remarkable anticipation despite his assumption that insects have spinal cords: 'But in less perfect animals, such as insects, whose cut off parts live, the animal spirits are primarily and immediately prepared not only in the brain, but also in the protuberances of the spinal marrow, or rather they are stored as in suitable repositaries, and hence it comes to pass that in the cut off portions of insects, the animal spirits are supplied for keeping up to some extent life and motions, from the small piece of spinal marrow connected with each portion.'[16]

Whytt's sympathy included what are now described as reflex actions: 'There is no sympathy between the different muscles or other parts of the body as was observed while the spinal marrow was entire; from whence it seems to follow that the nerves distributed to the several parts of the body have no communication but at their termination in the brain or spinal marrow, and to this perhaps, alone is owing the consent or sympathy between them.'[17]

[15] *Works*, p. 202.
[16] From Fearing, op. cit., p. 35.
[17] *Works*, p. 206.

Eckhard[18] regards this as the *Fundamentalversuch* of the experimental physiology of reflex action. It seems clear however that Preston was just as explicitly impressed with the importance of the nerve cord. In an 'Account of a child born without a brain',[19] he argued that the medulla spinalis generated, or filtered and distributed the animal spirits in the same way as the brain. He here also recalled the experiment of Duverney, who in 1673 took the cerebrum from a pigeon and filled the cranium with flax: it lived, searched for food, pursued the ordinary functions of life and had the use of sense, i.e. it responded to stimuli. This experiment, according to Baglivi, was well known, and certainly Whytt was acquainted with it.

Chirac showed by progressive destruction of the nervous system of a dog that the cerebellum was more essential to life than the cerebrum; but without the cerebellum, and even when the medulla oblongata is divided from the medulla spinalis, the dog could be sustained, with heart beat, by blowing air into the lungs.

The greatest discovery attributed to Whytt rests upon the following observation: 'A frog lives, and moves its members for half an hour after its head is cut off; nay, when the body of a frog is divided in two, both the anterior and posterior extremities preserve the life and power of motion for a considerable time.'[20]

Here, Whytt quotes not Hales, but Kaau: '*Impet. Faciens* No. 331'. Kaau is not mentioned by any modern author, although this passage is frequently quoted; it is held by Fearing to be the most important contribution of Whytt, whom he thought the most important figure in the history of reflex action up to his time. However, it must be owned that Whytt does not here specifically indicate that the lower extremity of the frog was sensible of irritations; according to his doctrine, it was alive, as it possessed soul, and the 'power of motion' could well apply to that proceeding spontaneously from the damaged nerve cord, or the motions produced when this was irritated: the irritation of the severed end of the medulla spinalis was not uncommon experimental practice. Thus while Whytt clearly recognized that only a section of the cord was necessary to originate motions, he does not make it clear in this paragraph whether this is a reflection of incoming impulses.

Caldani, performing experiments in 1764 at the request of Haller, cut a frog in half below the front legs, and observed that irritation of the rear legs caused them to move, i.e. this was a specific

[18] From Fearing, op. cit., p. 75.
[19] There are two similar papers in the same publication: Dr. Tyson, 'An infant with the brain depressed into the hollow of the vertebrae', *Phil. Trans.*, 1694-7, *19*, 533, and M. Bussière, 'Child born without a brain', *Phil. Trans.*, 1699, *21*, 141.
[20] *Works*, p. 203.

demonstration that only a segment of the cord was necessary for reflex action. Haller asked Caldani to observe any immobility from shock. Haller probably wanted this information for his dispute with Whytt, who had already demonstrated both shock and the segment-of-cord experiment.

Jefferson, for whom Whytt was 'by common consent, the greatest of the early neurophysiologists',[21] claimed that Whytt was the first to notice that the stretching of a muscle acts as a stimulus to its contraction. This was 'missed' by Marshall Hall. Jefferson adds that Whytt was 'shaky on the important issue of the unconscious nature of the reflex action...'. This seems remarkable, as Whytt's doctrines of vital and involuntary motions very specifically include the soul acting in an unconscious and obligatory way, and he was well aware of how this could go on in the absence of the conscious soul in the brain.

Thus it has been seen that different writers point to similar paragraphs taken from Whytt's work as 'fundamental' for the development of the reflex idea. These quotations refer to Whytt's undoubted wisdom in insisting on the importance of the spinal cord in certain involuntary motions but make no mention of Whytt's pointing out that only a segment of the cord was necessary. Canguilhem puts greater importance on Whytt's observation that shock persists for some fifteen minutes after decollation, temporarily destroying the power of the spinal cord to act as an organizing centre. He points to Whytt's experimental proof that all sympathy between the stimulated sense organ and the contracting muscle was owing to the spinal cord, since when the latter is destroyed, then the sympathy suffers a similar fate. He does not emphasize Whytt's remarks upon the divided spinal cord: 'Ici se place un exemple particulièrement important puisqu'il est un des premiers faits experimentaux mis en rapport avec la fonction de la moelle épinière dans la production des mouvements réflexes.'[22]

Fearing, however, does note that Whytt suggested that only a part of the cord was necessary for the reflex, but as has been observed, the quotation he chooses is open to objection.

It is argued here that the following quotation is more explicit: '. . . it must follow, that the motions and other signs of life which are observed in the body and limbs of a frog for above half an hour after its head is cut off, are to be attributed to the sentient principle,

[21] Sir Geoffrey Jefferson, 'Marshall Hall, the Grasp Reflex, and the Diastaltic Spinal Cord', Science, Medicine and History, Essays in Honour of Charles Singer, ed. E. A. Underwood, Oxford, 1953, vol. 2, p. 300.
[22] G. Canguilhem, La Formation du Concept de Réflexe aux xviie et xviiie Siècles, Paris, 1955, p. 102.

to which its motions were owing when in an entire state; and if so, then the motions of this body, when divided into two parts, must also be referred to the same cause, since they are of a like kind, though of shorter duration.'[23]

It refers to motions proceeding from the activity of the soul resident in the spinal cord both before and after decollation, and suggests the same mechanism is employed, since these motions *are of a like kind*: that is, such motions include those consequent upon a stimulus, as well as those arising spontaneously from the cord.

Thus although Fearing claims more for Whytt than Eckhard, or Singer and Underwood, and most other modern authors, they are generally agreed that the value of Whytt's work lies in his accurate observations and well-conceived experiments. The value Whytt placed upon observation may be a result of his early empirical training; it expressed itself in his admiration of Newton. This encouraged in him a scepticism of mechanical explanation which in turn led to a preconceived animism to which he held just as firmly as his contemporaries held to various kinds of mechanisms, but which did not in the least stand in the way of accurate interpretation of observation. Canguilhem[24] compares Astruc's use of the speculative concept of the reflex in a mechanistic explanation of his clinical observations, and Haller's support, from his encyclopedic knowledge of decapitated animals, of a neuromuscular conception bearing no relation to the reflex, with Whytt's experiments and clinical observations which supported an 'analyse anatomo-physiologique hostile à toute conjecture théorique, indifferente à toute systemisation'.[25]

Canguilhem describes the 'poverty'[26] of Whytt's theoretical concepts. By this he means the co-extension of the soul to all parts of the body; he observes that Whytt was obliged to do this in the light of his observations, and that the thought did not occur to him that there might be a multiplicity of organizing centres in the decapitated frog, rather than one extended. That Whytt did in fact consider this possibility is shown by recalling the attention he paid to the ideas of Alexander Stuart, for whom the terminations of the nerves were the 'brains' of the organ in which they occurred. Moreover, Whytt's ideas on the specific energies of nerves, the relationship between stimulus and response in quantity and quality and other elaborations of the laws he described which united body and soul, must be considered as part of his theoretical concepts, and which on this account, seem anything but poverty-stricken.

23 *Works*, p. 205.
24, 25 G. Canguilhem, op. cit., p. 101.
26 Ibid., p. 106.

The surprising fact is that Whytt, a confirmed animist, should have made possible a closer definition of the reflex, a motion as mechanical as any in the body. He did not use the term 'reflex' to mean anything but the power of self-knowledge, and even though his own sentient principle acted in an obligatory way, he disliked the term 'automatic' as suggesting the mechanical. (His opinion is expressed in a passage at the end of this chapter.) It is then, as Canguilhem[27] points out, precisely because Whytt did not co-operate in the development of the reflex idea that he is an interesting figure. What Whytt did do, and tried to do, was to show that the activities of the necessarily acting sentient principle tended towards the preservation of the organic whole; combined with his accuracy of procedure, this added another characteristic to the reflex act. One cannot but agree with Canguilhem: 'Son sens de la totalité organique et de l'insuffisance du mécanisme à en rendre compte, la liaison qu'il institue entre les mouvements réflexes et les instincts fondamentaux de conservation témoignent d'un grande esprit.'[28]

An important characteristic of the reflex, its speed of action, was clear to Whytt: '. . . the motions excited by pain or irritation are so instantaneous that there can be no time for the exercise of reason or comparison of ideas in order to their performance; but they seem to follow as a necessary and immediate consequence of the disagreeable perception'.[29]

This is an example of the quasi-mechanism typical of Whytt, and seems to be derived from animism and mechanism. Drawing the elements of his doctrine from both sets of ideas, he saw himself standing apart from both. Of mechanism he observed: 'Though perhaps there may be an impropriety in this term [automatic] as it may seem to convey the idea of a mere inanimate machine, producing such motions purely by value of its mechanical construction: a notion of the animal frame too low and absurd to be embraced by any but the most minute philosophers'.[30]

His refutation of the excessive animism of Stahl, expressed in similar terms, is given below, p.140.

Another important aspect of the reflex, that although beneficial, it is unlearned, was also known to Whytt: '. . . if we suppose our minds so formed and connected to our bodies, as that, in consequence of a stimulus affecting any organ or of an uneasy perception in it, they shall immediately excite such motions in this or that organ or part of the body as may be most proper to remove the

[27] Ibid., p. 101.
[28] Ibid., p. 106.
[29] *Works*, p. 151.
[30] *An Essay on the Vital and other Involuntary Motions of Animals*, p. 1.

irritating cause; and this without any previous conviction of such motions being necessary or conducive to this end.'[31]

These passages seem very distant from the contemporary protestations of Whytt's colleague Porterfield and other Stahlians, who claimed that even vital motions were once voluntary, and wise, and only by 'use or custom' became involuntary. Whytt everywhere insists on the necessary action of the soul according to laws and the original constitution of the body.

[31] *Works*, p. 151.

CHAPTER VIII

The Problem of the Seat of the Soul

We have already had some glimpses of Whytt's ideas on the nature and location of the soul. It was single. It was quite immaterial, and survived the death of the body. In the body it was responsible for all the manifestations of life: not only did it penetrate every part of the body, and restrict its activities according to the nature of that part which it occupied, but it also remained in the part for a short while after its excision from the body. Coextensive and divisible, (in this sense at least) it had one other great property, that in the body, apart from the brain, it was not a free agent, but was bound to act in accordance with certain laws.

Some of these ideas (singleness, immateriality and immortality) were the common property of the physicians and philosophers of the eighteenth century, the others not. The purpose of this chapter is to attempt to trace some of the historical reasons and antecedents of Whytt's unusual ideas, of which coextension is the primary. His physiological notions sprang from the idea of coextension, and it is of interest to follow the history of it and of its relationship to the opposing conception of a centralized or localized soul.

From the multitude of words used for, and the shades of meaning attached to the concept of 'soul', perhaps those are pre-eminent which express the idea that the soul is the cause of life. Life, in common parlance as among primitive peoples, is that which makes a creature move and breathe, which gives it heat, and endues it with sensations, and, if it be man, thought. Thought, sensation, heat, respiration and motion: five vital activities from which, in varying proportions, are compounded most conceptions of 'soul'.

Of these, respiration and sensation have been the most important. The manifest relationship between the behaviour of the heart and certain sudden and violent sensations, to say nothing of its activity in emotional states, led naturally to the conclusion that the heart was a centralized seat of the soul. For the Mesopotamian civilizations[1] the heart was the seat of intellect (yet emotion sprang from the liver, and cunning and compassion from the stomach and uterus) and the Egyptians took the greatest possible care in preserving

[1] K. D. Keele, op. cit., p. 6.

93

the heart of their dead,[2] for it was the earthly container of the immortal soul.

Respiration, the second of these two vital activities characteristic of a soul, must have had an influence upon the imagination equally as ancient and universal. The most obvious change attendant upon death is the cessation of breathing. Life and breath leave the body together: what more natural than that either or both of these should be identified with the soul? Many living primitive peoples believe in a 'breath soul',[3] and the importance of the inspired air was not lost upon the Egyptians: it was carried by the system of vessels which were associated with the sensory heart.[4]

The idea of the importance of air to life survived up to the seventeenth-century workers on respiration, and Whytt in the next century was unusual in believing that there was no *pabulam vitae* in air, seeming to dismiss this 'vivifying spirit'[5] as unnecessarily obscure.

The idea found its greatest expression in the early Greek idea of *pneuma*. The *pneuma* was the breath of life, drawn in from the surrounding air to the lungs, and from there to the blood and heart, vivifying the body and generating the psychic phenomena. We may see this in Homer,[6] where *thymos* is a vapour corresponding to the *pneuma*, lodged in the chest and lungs, and responsible for thought and sensation.[7] The *thymos* leaves the body at death, but does not itself survive. Personal immortality is assured by a second entity, the *psyche*. This is *not* conscious, nor, although it is 'breathed out' at death, is it the breath-soul, but is identified with the person and located in his head. It survives in Hades. Again then, the heart is the *central* organ, as with the Egyptians, the seat of intellect and emotions and here associated with the breath of life; while the *pneuma*, carried by the blood to all parts, was coextensive with the body. Like the Babylonians, Homer speaks of other organs, the liver and diaphragm, as further centres of emotion.[8] The location of the *psyche* in the head gives the first glimmer of the importance that organ was to assume in later philosophies, while the *material* co-

[2] Ibid., p. 5.

[3] Sir J. Frazer, *The Golden Bough*, London, 1925, (abridged ed.) p. 180.

[4] K. D. Keele, op.cit., p. 4.

[5] *Works*, p. 31.

[6] Professor Onions, *Origins of Greek and Roman Thought*, Cambridge. (Quoted by F. M. Cornford, *Plato's Cosmology*, London, 1937, p. 284.)

[7] M. D. Altschule, 'The pneuma concept of the soul', *J. Hist. Behav. Sci.*, 1965, *1*, 315.

[8] D. H. M. Woollam, 'Concepts of the Brain and its Functions in Classical Antiquity', *The History and Philosophy of Knowledge of the Brain and its Functions* ed. F. N. L. Poynter, Oxford, 1958, p. 7.

extension of the *pneuma* or soul was an idea which lasted long enough to be attacked by Whytt.

That mere matter could initiate motion was as absurd to Whytt (at the head of whose essay on the motions of animals stands a quotation from Cicero to the effect that only that which is self-moving has a soul) as it was to Thales, the first of the Milesian philosophers. For him, the essence of the soul was its power to move itself: man, animals and the lodestone were the possessors of souls. Further, all objects of nature were created from water, in which life was inherent. All things were alive by their very nature and nothing more so than animals, every portion of them having its soul.[9] This kind of view was held by Anaximenes, also of Miletus. Here the *pneuma*[10] or air was the common stuff of the universe: the basic elemental material from which all 'physical' things and the *psyche*[11] were made, the breath which, coextensive with the body and holding it together, also held together the universe, and admitted no strict distinction between the two.

Pythagoras introduced the idea (either from his teacher Pherecydes or his travels to Egypt) that the soul was immortal. *Pneuma*[12] is again drawn in from the air and its vital activities associated with the heart. The brain seems to have been the seat of the 'mind' rather than the 'soul',[13] perhaps in the way that Homer described. Other features of this immortal soul were paralleled by the Christian conception of the soul.

In none of these ancient ideas can we press too close a comparison to later conceptions. We know of Anaximenes through his single surviving sentence, and of Pythagoras largely by way of his disciples. It is impossible to say whether the *psyche*, *thymos* and *pneuma* were aspects of a soul as single as that favoured in the eighteenth century, but extended through the body; or how the faculties of the soul were related to the body, as in Whytt's very explicit statement. In many cases we must be content to discover the location of the faculties of the soul, observing however, that this can sometimes be an unsatisfactory guide to the seat of the soul itself.

The Greek philosophers of the fifth century developed these ideas. The *pneuma* remained associated with a sensory heart, and the matter from which it was made became, in the views of different

[9] B. Farrington, *Greek Science*, Penguin Books, 1961, p. 37.
[10] H. Diels, *Fragmente der Vorsokratiker*, 7th ed., Berlin, 1954-6, chap. 13. (Quoted by L. J. Rather, 'G. E. Stahl's psychological physiology', *Bull. Hist. Med.*, 1961, 35, 37.
[11] H. E. Sigerist, *A History of Medicine*, New York, 1961, vol. 2, p. 92.
[12] M. D. Altschule, op. cit., p. 315.
[13] H. E. Sigerist, op. cit., p. 99.

schools of thought, either atomic or elementary; consisting, that is, of 'elements', the most notable of which had been the air of Anaximenes. The *pneuma* which for Heraclitus was the highest, intelligent, life principle, by which man breathes in divine reason, was also an element, fire. Clearly fire, particularly when conceived as a universal ether,[14] is the most suited of all natural substances to be the soul, on account of its subtlety, its rapidity of motion, and near approach to what must seem to be immateriality. To air, the contemporary Parmenides added earth, so that now the soul, with two elements, was distinct from the *pneuma*, which could hardly include earth in its composition. The distinction was emphasized by Parmenides' strict regard for what was animate and what was inanimate in nature: no ambient air could be soul, or alive, nor could it produce inorganic nature, as it had for Anaximenes.[15] The new soul remained centralized in the heart.

Empedocles went further. In line with the rest of his philosophy, the soul was made up from the four elements, earth, air, fire and water. Sensation was effected by each element perceiving[16] its counterpart in the outside world, and this (according to Aristotle)[17] Empedocles equated with thinking. This perceiving soul, the organ of consciousness, was seated in the blood of the heart.[18] Although the *pneuma* seems to have been left behind, just as in the case of Parmenides, it was in fact revived among the followers of Empedocles.

Before following the other developments of the *pneuma* idea into atomism, where the theory may be said to have come into full flower, we must take note of a parallel development of a quite different character. With Alcmaeon of Croton, we seem to move suddenly nearer to the eighteenth century. Possibly taking a hint from his master Pythagoras, Alcmaeon firmly placed the soul in the brain.[19] Dissecting out the optic nerves, he concluded that as the eyes were the organs of vision, so was the faculty of seeing (and of other senses) located in the brain. Here, too, were thought and memory, and, although the senses had different localizations, a sensorium, the place (or faculty) common to all senses and a term of some importance in the problem of the seat of the soul.

[14] M. D. Altschule, op. cit., p. 314.
[15] R. O. Moon, *Hippocrates and his Successors in Relation to the Philosophy of Their Time*, London, 1923, pp. 55-61, 81.
[16] H. E. Sigerist, op. cit., p. 108.
[17] Aristotle, *Complete Works*, ed. J. A. Smith and W. D. Ross, Oxford, 1908-52, vol 3, *De Anima*, bk. 3, 427a.
[18] H. M. Brown, 'The anatomical habitat of the soul', *Ann. Med. Hist.*, 1923, 5, 1.
[19] H. E. Sigerist, op. cit., p. 102.

Alcmaeon was supported by Anaxagoras, who in addition said that the mind of man was a distinct improvement over the condition of animals, which had a soul only. Anaxagoras' cosmogony involved Mind organizing a Chaos of the particulate seeds of future existence, and is thought to have anticipated the atomic theories of Leucippus and Democritus. Democritus also followed Alcmaeon, possibly accepting the same Pythagoreanism through his teacher Philolaus, who, (the first to write of Pythagoras) held that the mind was in the brain, but the soul in the heart. This distinction is not alone: there were four vital organs, brain, heart, navel and genitalia, and the mind was seated in the brain, the soul and sensation in the heart, growth of the embryo in the navel and procreation in the genitalia.[20] This recognition of nervous, animal and vegetative functions foreshadows that of Plato and Aristotle.

With Democritus himself we return to atomism, with the associated importance of *pneuma* and the brain, which flourished until demolished by Aristotle. The atoms of the soul were the atoms of fire, small, smooth and spherical. Normally moving with the external air, as a true *pneuma*, they were drawn into the body during respiration, and distributed over the body by the blood. Whytt drew upon some aspects of ancient atomism to substantiate his own idea of a coextensive soul, and both systems of animism have some common characteristics: coextension was essential, as neither of them could conceive that matter was alive unless in the presence of a soul. Whytt also followed Democritus in the idea that the soul had different functions in the parts to which it stretched.[21] This is the natural consequence of a coextensive soul, when all the appearances of life are believed to come from the soul, as both authors held, and Democritus differs in placing anger in the heart and desire in the liver, ideas codified by Plato. The atoms of the soul insinuate themselves one between every two atoms of the body, initiate motion by drawing these two atoms after them, and are dispersed randomly after death. Such materiality and mortality were repugnant to the eighteenth-century mind, but Whytt would have agreed that the reasoning part of the soul (by a concentration of atoms, said Democritus) is seated in the brain, yet having the power of sentience throughout the body like Whytt's sentient principle.

A synthesis of some of these ideas was effected in the eclectic philosophy of Diogenes of Apollonia. The *pneuma* is again in evidence: it is air, like that of Anaximenes, and intelligent, as was Heraclitus' ether. This *pneuma* entered the body of the otherwise

[20] Ibid., p. 99.
[21] R. O. Moon, op. cit., p. 81.

97

inanimate infant at the moment of birth (a point disputed until the time of Whytt) and, reaching the lungs, was distributed all over the body. Coextension of this kind was more necessary to a material soul, as with Democritus, than with the immaterial soul of Whytt, although for the same reasons: to give life to matter by its immediate presence. Distributing heat and life over the body by means of the blood, the *pneuma* was nevertheless specialized in function in one part of the body; retaining its airy nature in the vessels around the brain, it was responsible for sensation. The soul itself was in the air inside the brain.[22]

In this way, during the fifth century, the brain rivalled the heart as the organ and seat of sensation (which was not necessarily coincident with the seat of the soul). This dichotomy of opinion is well illustrated in the Hippocratic body of writings. The author of the treatise *On the Heart* uncomprisingly places air, the seat of innate heat and the intelligence which controls the soul, in the left ventricle.[23] The book *Diseases of Maidens* suggests the same, while in *On the Sacred Disease*, the brain is put forward as the centre of sensation, consciousness and emotion.[24] Depending on the interpretation of the authorship of these works, then, either the brain is the organ used by the soul, given the power of intelligence by the air, which first reaches and leaves its essence here, or the right ventricle of the heart, sending blood to the lungs, is more closely related to the *pneuma* tradition. This ventricle receives air in exchange from the lungs, and this air, contained alone only in the *left* ventricle, fulfills all the duties of the soul.

Passing on to the fourth century, we come to two authors of great importance to later philosophy and science, Plato and Aristotle. For the first time we have a complete account of the soul, and can be sure, in considering its details, that they have a direct influence on Western thought of many centuries later. The assimilation of neoplatonism by early Christianity contributed to the climate of theological ideas from which Whytt drew, while Aristotle's influence on all philosophy need not be emphasized.

Man, said Plato, has an immortal and a mortal soul. The immortal soul, rational and perceptive, was created by the demiurge and placed in the part of man nearest heaven, the head.[25] The similarity to the Christian soul, created by God, is clear. To it,

[22] K. D. Keele, op. cit., p. 18.
[23] H. Sigerist, op. cit., pp. 274, 325.
[24] W. Penfield, 'Hippocratic Preamble: the Brain and Intelligence', *The History and Philosophy of Knowledge of the Brain and its Functions*, ed. F. N. L. Poynter, Oxford, 1958, p. 3.
[25] F. M. Cornford, *Plato's Cosmology*, London, 1937, p. 150.

Plato added the mortal soul which was formed with the body by the inferior deities. There is an unexpected parallel between this and Whytt's idea that God created purely immaterial 'intelligences', and that animals derived the faculties of their souls (corresponding to Plato's mortal soul) from these.

Part of the lower soul described by Plato was concerned with anger and associated conditions and placed in the heart, and part with concupiscence, in the liver.[26] This plurality of souls was undesirable to later Christian philosophers, and much of the later history of the concept of the soul centred around the adoption of all these characteristics by a single soul.

The contributions of Plato to science are disputed among historians, and it cannot be denied here that, however much they were later taken as scientific, these speculations of Plato are more nearly related to his political notions of 'rational', 'brave' and 'concupiscent' groups of citizens, than to scientific observations of the sort, for example, of which Aristotle was capable.

Many historical threads come together in Plato, and are passed on by him to Aristotle and the philosophic tradition of the West. The immortality of the soul[27] is of course an older idea. Plato's friend Architas Tarentinus was as much convinced of this Pythagorean idea as Plato himself and passed on the (for Plato) germinal ideas that the mind was located in the brain and soul in the heart, which we have met in the teachings of his master Philolaus. In speaking of the 'spirited' soul in the heart, that which was the fount of anger, courage and loyalty, Plato uses the word *thymos*,[28] which links up at once with the *pneuma* tradition. The lungs exist to cool the heart, an idea taken over by Aristotle, who did not associate it with *pneuma*. He did, however, use a kind of *pneuma* to explain inheritance, and which was therefore present in the semen. By a similar argument Plato derived the soul in the semen from the spinal cord and brain, imagining that the card was connected to the organs of generation.[29] Aristotle's idea may derive from Hippocrates, who had said that as the semen was the only substance passed from generation to generation, it must be almost entirely soul, which was therefore more nearly water than blood.

Again, in using *psyche* for the soul in the head, Plato seems to be using the Homeric or Pythagorean tradition, having transferred to this *psyche* the powers of reason of the older soul (in the heart). The

[26] Plato, *Timaeus*, trans. J. Warrington, London, 1965, p. 38.
[27] P. Friedländer, *Plato. An Introduction*, trans. H. Meyerhoff, London, 1958, p. 183.
[28] F. M. Cornford, op. cit., p. 284.
[29] K. D. Keele, op. cit., p. 27.

atomism employed by Plato, and the mechanism he envisaged whereby the soul perceived the external counterparts of its own structure are further ideas with historical antecedents.

Some of these ideas were taken by Aristotle and welded together with his own into a convincing whole. The concupiscent soul which Plato had put in the liver, at the furthest remove from the rational soul, was replaced[30] by Aristotle with the nutritive soul. This was an inherent property of living matter, enabling it to feed and grow, and so was not only in the liver, but was coextensive. Plants had this but no other powers. Animals, in addition, had a sensitive capacity corresponding to the spirited soul of Plato, and it was by means of this that they could react to their surroundings. Like Whytt's 'sentient principle', the sensitive soul did *not* include the power of conscious perception in these circumstances. Man alone possessed this power, the attribute of his unique soul, the rational. This itself suffered a division into two parts, the imaginative and the appetitive. Further, there was a distinction between mind and soul: the mind was independently implanted in the soul (without spatial distinction), and was that whereby the soul thinks and judges, a form capable of appreciating forms, and the means by which the appetitive soul initiated motion.

Of these distinctions, the threefold division of the soul of man, nutritive, sentient, rational, remained the most important. Yet these were not three different souls, but rather each successive soul was an elaboration of the one which went before, and all remained a single whole in man. Now, whereas what we shall call for convenience the nutritive soul shared two characteristics with Whytt's soul, that it was a kind of vital force which enabled matter to live, assimilate food and grow, and (as it was the form of the matter) that it was indisseverable from that matter and thus coextensive with the body, it did, nevertheless, have a principal location. This was the heart. Here, food, midway between the point of its entry and that of its expulsion, reached the most intense stage of its metabolism, and this, the concern of the nutritive soul, was accompanied by a correspondingly great degree of heat, the invariable companion of this soul. (In a similar way Whytt, unlike most of his contemporaries, insisted that animal heat, impossible to explain on mechanical principles, was the product of the soul and absolutely necessary to its two prime functions, sensibility and irritability.)

Other evidence also pointed to the importance of the heart. Of all the organs, the heart was the first to make its embryological

---

[30] G. S. Claghorn, *Aristotle's Criticism of Plato's 'Timaeus'*, The Hague, 1954, p. 67.

appearance, performing the nutritive faculty for the remainder; its heat was not only essential for life, but as the source of bodily heat, had a critical low point, below which, unlike the other organs, it could not be safely cooled. Here, too, was the sensitive soul. The dependence of this on the nutritive soul made it reasonable that it should be found where the latter had its principal seat, and the manifest reaction of the heart to external disturbances and internal states of mind, as anger or joy, clearly indicated that it was to this point that all the impressions from the sense organs were directed: this was the origin of the nerves, the *sensorium commune*.

The rational soul, said Aristotle in *De Respiratione*,[31] was equally dependent on the power of nutrition and its natural fire, but relating not at all to matter, its immateriality denied it either extension or locality. While these characteristics of the three souls (for convenience thinking of them as separate entities) seem to differ widely from those of Whytt's sentient principle (and of course, the shift of the *sensorium* to the brain is a profound change), an observation made by Aristotle of a very much more down-to-earth nature inclined him to relate the three souls more closely together. It was precisely the same observation which led Whytt into his speculations on the extension and characteristics of the soul. In this observation of nature the two sets of ideas seem more closely related.

The observation was this: 'It is a fact of observation that plants and certain insects go on living when divided into segments: this means that each of the segments has a soul in it identical in species, though not numerically identical in the different segments, for both the segments for a time possess the power of sensation and local motion'.[32]

Whytt, it may be recalled, equally thought that an excised organ contained the soul in the same way as it did in the body, i.e. limited by the tissue that contained it. The division of an animal into two living segments in this way raises the vexed question of the divisibility of the soul: was this extended soul of Whytt's doctrine divided in this process? Was, indeed, that of Aristotle? Whytt claimed that the immateriality of the soul precluded division, but he did not fully meet the objection that it would also preclude extension. Aristotle escaped this particular difficulty as the rational soul did not have extension among its properties (being immaterial), and anyway was not possessed by an insect. In general, he said, the

[31] Aristotle, *Complete Works*, vol. 3, *De Somniis*, 474b.
[32] Ibid., *De Anima*, 411b.

soul was not divisible into its parts but was divisible as a whole. Divisible, that is, as his translator observes, 'in a sense, i.e., so as to preserve its homogeneity even in its smallest part'.[33]

Each part of the divided insect, then, contained both parts of the soul and the souls so present in each part are homogeneous with each other, and with the whole: in a word, the soul is coextensive with the body. The difficulties Whytt ran into over the coextensive soul he described stemmed from the fact that it was a soul adopted from one which had evolved from Aristotle's by the fusion of the original three souls to produce one which was single. Whereas Aristotle escaped Whytt's problems by treating each soul separately, Whytt had to explain a soul that was immaterial for theological reasons, extended to meet physiological needs and indivisible in the face of anatomical appearance. The spiritual and immaterial soul was incompatible with the physical processes it had to engage in and which it had inherited from Aristotle.

Thus Aristotle firmly re-established the heart as the seat of the soul. Despite doubts expressed by his pupils, like Theophrastus (and Zenocrates, who favoured the brain),[34] this became the orthodox view. It was assented to by the atomists and in particular Epicurus, who nevertheless disagreed with Aristotle in almost every other particular. The atoms of the soul were the round atoms of fire, in good Democritean tradition, dispersed through the body and unable to remain together outside it.

After Aristotle the scene shifts to Alexandria, where the two anatomists Herophilus and Erasistratus had considerable knowledge of the nervous system (unlike Aristotle) and unhesitatingly centralized the seat of the soul in the brain. Herophilus is credited with being the first to describe the ventricles of the brain, and it has long been believed that this is where he put the soul; it is more correct however to regard these cavities as the site where the powers relating to all activities were put into play, the soul itself residing in the substance of the base of the brain.[35] His fourth ventricle was particularly important as it was close to the spinal cord and motor nerves.[36] Although conditions in Alexandria made human dissection possible, Herophilus' brain anatomy is largely derived from the ox.[37] Erasistratus at first disagreed with Herophilus, and put the

[33] In a footnote to *De Anima*, 411b.
[34] H. M. Brown, op. cit., p. 8.
[35] W. Pagel, 'Medieval and Renaissance Contributions to the Knowledge of the Brain and its Functions', *The History and Philosophy of Knowledge of the Brain and its Functions*, ed. F. N. L. Poynter, Oxford, 1958, p. 95.
[36] K. D. Keele, op. cit., p. 41.
[37] D. H. Woollam, op. cit., p. 12.

soul in the meninges,[38] which he thought were the origin of the nerves. Later he considered the soul to be in the cerebellum, and so did not differ too seriously from his fellow Alexandrian, although he also held that the intelligence of man could be attributed to the richness of the cortical convolutions of the cerebral hemispheres. It was probably his influence upon his contemporary, Strato, that made the latter place the soul in that part of the brain behind the eyebrows.[39]

The *pneuma* idea was not lost, even to Herophilus, for whom the arteries contained *pneuma zotikon*, or vital spirit, transmitted from the heart to the flesh. The idea that the *pneuma* was something less than, or a servant to the soul was elaborated in this way by Galen. A more old-fashioned *pneuma* was accepted by Cleanthes:[40] from a universal vivifying ether, it pervaded the entire body. His pupil Chrysippus developed the idea in an interesting way, combining several older notions. The *pneuma*, as soul, entered into total union[41] with all parts of the body, and like other coextensive souls, but more explicitly, its function in every part was related to that part: it saw in the eyes, tasted in the tongue, and heard in the ears. The ability to feel was spread all over the body, as with the coextensive souls of the atomists, and of Whytt. Yet the soul had its principal seat in the heart, where these faculties *conveniunt*.[42] Chrysippus said the Platonic and Aristotelian concupiscent (vegetative) and irascible (sentient) faculties were identical, so that the soul had two faculties only, the rational and irrational.[43] Interestingly, Chrysippus speaks of 'common sense' (*sensus communis* in the sixteenth-century version of Galen) as that sense common to all men rather than that common to all senses.[44] This is more or less the modern meaning of the phrase, to which it returned after a digression in the middle ages.

The concept of *pneuma* became complex with the Stoics (of whom Chrysippus was one) and in that it often involved a coextensive soul, we may look at it a little more closely. Generally *pneuma* was a very tenuous substance spread through the body. Its function was to organize matter into several states of complexity, and so, producing material effects, it had itself to be material: it was

[38] H. M. Brown, op. cit., p. 9.
[39] K. D. Keele, op. cit., p. 41.
[40] H. M. Brown, op. cit., p. 6.
[41] S. Toulmin and J. Goodfield, *The Architecture of Matter*, Pelican Books, 1965, p. 107.
[42] Galen, *De Hippocratis et Platonis Placitis*, Paris, 1534, p. 21.
[43] Galen, op. cit., pp. 73, 81.
[44] Ibid., p. 21.

composed of varying proportions of fire and air, each related to its function. Thus the highest *pneuma* was pure fire, the substance of the outer heavens, immortal and conferring intelligence on man. Less highly organized matter required as its guiding principle *pneuma* with a greater complement of air, and in this way the vital *pneuma* animated the body while the lowest, cohesive *pneuma* was responsible for the unity of the body and the fixed pattern of properties characteristic of its raw materials.[45]

These different states of *pneuma*, like the divisions of the Aristotelian soul, were not necessarily distinct from each other. A physical basis was needed to explain the action of the *psyche* which was the cause of every organized state, and the *pneuma*, satisfying this need, was simply an aspect of the *psyche*. Probably Moschion, in the next century, had these kinds of reasons for placing the soul throughout the body. The Stoics influenced the Eclectic school of philosophy in the first century before Christ, yet they (if eclecticism can be reconciled with unanimity) generally retained the heart as the principal seat of the soul. Even Peripatetics such as Critolaus were adherents of a *pneuma* theory. Another, non-pneumatist follower of Aristotle, Poseidonius, is only worthy of note to avoid confusion with another later author of the same name.

Lucretius (first century B.C.) advocated the kind of coextensive soul we have already met in the atomism of Democritus and Epicurus, whose system Lucretius expounded. The mind, distinct from the remainder of the soul in this at least, resided in the heart, the destination of sensation and origin of motion. It may be assumed that Whytt was familiar with the poem, *De Rerum Natura*, for he quotes Lucretius in support of his own interpretation of this point, that is, that there is no real distinction between soul and mind: 'Nunc animum, atque animam dico conjuncta teneri Inter se, atque unam naturam conficere ex se' (Book 3, line 137).

Whytt wisely does not extend the quotation, for the poem continues to explain that not only is the *animus*, the mind, located in the heart, but also, just like the *anima*, is composed of matter. However much Whytt would have disagreed with this, he may not have been uninfluenced by the preceding part of the poem which describes how the *anima*, spread out to and enlivening all parts of the body, remains for a short time in a limb which may happen to be cut off. Later, the correspondence with Whytt's ideas becomes more marked: the *anima* suffers division with its body, as can be seen when a limb severed in battle writhes on the ground. Further, Lucretius was as impressed as Whytt (and Aristotle with his insects)

[45] S. Toulmin and J. Goodfield, op. cit., p. 102.

that each part freshly cut from a living snake continues alive for some time. All three authors decided that the soul must be present in each of the parts, but only Lucretius took it as evidence of the mortality of the soul.

Animus, which Lucretius uses as the equivalent of *mens* (mind), corresponds to the *psyche* of the Greeks, while *anima* here is variously the counterpart of *pneuma* or *thymos*. There is, running through all these terms, the idea of a higher and lower, or hierarchy of souls, as we have seen in Aristotle. The *pneuma* tradition appears very strongly in Lucretius, both *animus* and *anima* being aspects of the same 'breath'. This 'mind stuff' consists of small round atoms of air and 'rarefied wind', to which are added heat and a nameless fourth substance of even finer atoms, the ultimate mysterious life-giving element. The atoms of these substances, very much smaller than those proposed by Democritus, swirl about over the body creating a single, living substance. The body enters into this creation, for while mind is latent over all the body, it is only by interaction of body and the atoms of soul that sentience can come into being. This absolute dependence of mind on matter recalls Whytt's notion that the soul relied for its local characteristics on the matter in which it subsisted. Away from these organs, the body, it lost all characteristics save that of its continued existence. For Lucretius, it lost this too. If the soul were immortal, he argued, then it should possess its properties, particularly consciousness, in the absence of matter and during immortality. We should have memories of former existences, we should use the body as if it were a house, and not be limited in perception by ageing and inefficient sense organs. All this Lucretius refutes in a passage sufficiently similar to Whytt's elegant rejection of Nicholls (p. 140) (who had postulated a soul similarly independent of matter) that it is difficult not to find Whytt's inspiration in it. What evidence is there, asks Lucretius, that souls search out body-atoms and construct dwelling places for themselves? 'When the dwelling is weakened by age, does the soul wish to escape from inside? Is it afraid to remain in an ageing and mouldering lodging, afraid its house might collapse? Surely no immortal soul need fear such danger.'[46]

Lucretius dismisses the ideas of those who held that the soul was no more than a harmony of the bodily parts and senses. Previous writers like Aristoxenus and Dicearchus had said this,[47] and something of the sort was held by Lucretius' older contemporary

[46] Lucretius, *De Rerum Natura*, ed. S. Havercamp, Basle, 1725, vol. I, bk. III v. 770.
[47] A. Behrens, *Considerationem Animae Rationalis Medicam*, Leipzig, 1720, p. 5.

Asclepiades, who, moreover, made experiments to prove it: observing that various animals showed evidence of intelligence after the removal of their hearts or brains, he concluded that there could be no such thing as a soul as normally understood.

So far we have seen that the soul as conceived by Whytt has some relationship to that of Aristotle on one hand and the atomists, particularly Democritus, on the other. Its other essential ingredient, immortality, and the associated condition of immateriality, derives from the rise of Christian thought, to which our survey now brings us. From the decay of ancient science only the *pneuma* idea of the soul seems to have survived in any vigour. For the Pneumatist sect of physicians, founded in Rome in the first century by Athenaeus,[48] the *pneuma* was not only the soul and the cause of diseases, but was related to a deity who was the creator of men. Similarly the early Christians, like St. Luke, the physician, thought of the immortal soul as *pneuma*. The authority of the Old Testament decreed that this soul was in the heart; St. Matthew was among the first to mention this as a Christian tradition. Perhaps this, like the older *pneuma*, was related to the ether of the highest regions, for we are told that exceedingly holy persons were rendered light to the point of levitation by its kinship with heaven. Not least among these was St. Joseph of Copertino who flew about over the heads of his onlookers uttering 'his customary shrill cries'.

However, *pneuma* finds no place in the *Onomasticon* of Pollux, written in the second century A.D. Pollux lists many opinions of the ancients as regards the seat of the soul, and adopts a Platonic division of the soul with seats in the brain, heart and liver.[49] The *Onomasticon* was a useful work of reference in the West, and its list of authors with their views turns up in many medieval works on the seat of the soul. The relevant material probably comes from Soranus, a physician of slightly earlier date.

Also depending largely on Soranus is the similar compilation in the *De Anima* of Tertullian,[50] completed in 207. Apart from this, however, Tertullian is original. As a defender of the new Church, and a source of much Christian literature, he surprisingly makes the soul material. Immortal it certainly is, but its distinct origin in time (it is generated with the body) distinguishes it from the soul described by Plato and other pagan philosophers. It is a sort of immortal *pneuma*, not, indeed, bearing such a name, being derived from the breath of God Himself, but in other respects similar to it:

---

[48] M. D. Altschule, op. cit., p. 318.
[49] J. Pollux, *Onomasticon*, Amsterdam, 1706, vol. I, bk. 2, pp. 226-31.
[50] Tertullian, *De Anima*, ed. J. H. Waszink, Amsterdam, 1947.

in function it is the *spiritus*, the life-breath, and the mind; it is coextensive with the body and has an 'airy' colour. The faculty of Mind, on the evidence of the Scriptures, is located in the heart, (Asclepiades being dismissed), but the power of sentience[51] is in all parts of the flesh, as with Whytt's, and other coextensive souls. The soul originates and is given its sex with the body from the two components of the sperm, *humor*, corporeal and derived from the flesh of Adam, and *calor*, psychic, from the breath of God. The soul seems to linger a while in the body after what appears to be death. We may recall that certain appearances of life after 'death' brought Whytt to the same opinion.

Meanwhile the work of Herophilus and Erasistratus had been discovered and enlarged by Galen. Galen does not have a lot to say on the soul, but shows the influence of Plato and Hippocrates. The soul is located in the substance of the brain,[52] which could be shown quite clearly to be the origin of the nerves, the organs of sense and motion. Its immediate agent was the psychic *pneuma* in the ventricles[53] of the brain and the nerves. Soft sensory nerves arose from the front of the brain, in the substance of which were the sensory faculties; correspondingly, hard motor nerves sprang from the back of the brain, where the more rigid brain structure was suited to the function of memory.[54] The material psychic *pneuma*, or animal spirit, was elaborated from the vital spirit, and this from the animal spirit. This threefold division reflects the hierarchies of faculties of Plato and Aristotle, but here they are strictly the agents of the soul. Employing the familiar argument that there can be no interaction between matter and a supposedly immaterial soul, Galen concluded that the *psyche* was material and mortal.

With Galen we effectively come to the end of ancient science, and may pause to survey some of the origins of animism. Animism, the idea that all the phenomena of life spring from the presence of a soul, was almost universal; but explaining these phenomena in animals and man was not necessarily the same as explaining consciousness and the mental faculties in man alone. As a result there often arose another principle, supposed to be immortal and immaterial, and sometimes seated in a particular part of the body. Correspondingly the 'lower' principle was frequently conceived to be material and mortal, and often coextensive with the body it vivified. Such systems we have met with Homer, Pythagoras, Plato and Aristotle. The undesirability of accepting more than one principle led later to

[51] Tertullian uses *sensus communis* in the same way as Chrysippus.
[52] Galen, *De Hippocratis et Platonis Dogmatibus*, Basle, 1550, book 8, cap. I.
[53] W. Pagel, op. cit., p. 98.
[54] Galen, *De Usu Partium Corporis Humani*, Paris, 1528, p. 272.

attempts to attribute all the necessary characteristics to one soul.

From a mixture of these ideas developed the climate of opinion from which Whytt drew his concepts. His particular notion that the soul was coextensive was matched most readily by the atomists, from whom he drew, and secondly from those who thought the soul was single and immaterial. An immaterial soul can have no dimension and cannot be related physically to matter: it cannot have location in the body. As its effects are manifest in the body, some relationship had to be found between the two. It was decided the soul was related *illocaliter* to the body, as an Aristotelian form was related to its matter. It was thus 'formally' or 'virtually' present in all parts of the body, in a kind of immaterial coextension. The Platonists and neoplatonists of late antiquity and early middle ages seem to have favoured this interpretation. The scholastics took it over in the form *tota in toto et tota in qualibet parte totius*: the whole soul is in the whole body and wholly in any part of it. Whytt defended himself against charges of divisibility and extension of the soul by quoting these arguments.

The assimilation of neoplatonism by Christianity, and the influence of Plato himself made the early Christian writers (whose attention was naturally drawn to the immortal, rational soul) uncertain as to its seat. On the one hand the brain was indicated by Plato, and on the other, the heart by Aristotle and the Old Testament. Perhaps an answer was found in the 'formal' relationship of body and soul in the neoplatonism of Plotinus and Porphyry. During this time, too, the influence of Aristotle diminished until knowledge of his writings was lost to the West at the fall of the Roman Empire, the church alone continuing with its own selection of ancient culture.

Thus, in the fourth century, while such a stalwart of the Church as St. Jerome located the soul in the heart, another Church Father, St. Ambrose, was more neoplatonic, and Lactantius[55] apparently employed both heart and brain. There was an answer to that, too, which was used increasingly, particularly when Galen came to be a greater authority even than Plato: the soul was rooted in the heart and manifest only in the brain, where it performed its operations.

[55] H. M. Brown, op. cit., p. 12.

CHAPTER IX

The Ventricular Theory: a Digression

In following the history of the problem of the seat of the soul, we are inevitably led through that medieval episode when the ventricles of the brain were considered to be the seat of some of the faculties of the soul. The links between this and Whytt's animism are tenuous and indirect, but to omit any reference to the theory would be to give quite a wrong impression of the evolution of a concept.

Tenuous and indirect, the links are nevertheless there, and the inception and subsequent disappearance of the ventricular theory left at the end of the middle ages a significance of the word 'soul' different from that attached to it in late antiquity. The first appearance of the ventricular theory seems to be in the works of Poseidonius[1] of Byzantium, who studied the results of brain injury. Should the anterior part of the brain be damaged then so would the *phantastikon*, the proper recording of sensual perception, whereas the posterior portion controlled memory. This much he in all probability took from Galen who had said just the same. Poseidonius, however, concluded that reason was located *inside* the middle ventricle. This seems to have been developed by Nemesius, Bishop of Emesus,[2] shortly afterwards. Perception was placed in the anterior ventricles, reason in the middle and memory in the posterior ventricle.[3] Nemesius also speaks of the effects of wounds on the different ventricles, showing his probable debt to Poseidonius.

It would be too facile to imagine that Nemesius was putting the soul in the brain, and that these were its divisions, for, like a good Christian, he regarded the soul as single, immaterial and incapable of being localized: the ventricles were its organs, containing its faculties. This may be Christian neoplatonism,[4] for non-Christian neoplatonists, like Macrobius in the next century, put the soul in the brain and its spirits in the ventricles. It was at all events a kind of Platonism. Chalcidius translated Plato's *Timaeus* in this century, and contributed further to the non-dimensional relationship of

---

[1] W. Pagel, op. cit., p. 97.
[2] Ibid., p. 99.
[3] Nemesius, *The Nature of Man*, trans. G. Wither, London, 1636, p.335.
[4] W. Pagel, op. cit., p. 103.

109

body and soul. Effectively, the soul was present in all parts of the body.

This point of view was taken up for the Church by St. Augustine also; he suggested the posterior ventricle was the seat of motion, while memory resided in the middle ventricle.[5] He notes also the reference in the psalms[6] to the soul in the heart and concludes with his contemporary Nemesius, that the immaterial soul cannot be localized. St. Augustine's influence outweighed Tertullian's; the soul was not material, but they agreed it was generated with the body and was single. Its names, said St. Augustine, were as legion as its faculties. It was the *spiritus* in contemplation, *animus* in knowing, *mens* in understanding, *anima* in vivifying, *ratio* in choosing and *memoria* and *voluntas* in memory and will.[7] No more complete fusion of the old Platonic hierarchy of souls could be achieved.

The neoplatonic version of the body-soul relationship was furthered in the fifth century by Proclus and in the sixth by St. Remigius and Simplicius, who gave a neoplatonic interpretation to Aristotle's *De Anima*. Aëtius the Byzantine continued the tradition of putting the mental faculties in the ventricles of the brain.

The ventricular theory by now had moved east; the West depended for its knowledge of the soul on the work of encyclopedists summarizing classical knowledge. Thus while the earliest medieval writers had put the soul in the heart on biblical authority, the encyclopedist Isidore of Seville in the seventh century located it in the brain, under the influence of fragments of Plato, and neoplatonism. Macrobius and Chalcidius' translation of the *Timaeus* have already been mentioned. The ninth-century encyclopedist Hrabanus Maurus held similar ideas.[8]

Costa ben Lucca was another ninth-century compiler, and it seems that the Arabic elaboration of the ventricle theory can be traced back to him. Poseidonius and Aëtius were of Byzantium, as was Theophilus who in the seventh century put the faculties in the substance of the brain corresponding to the ventricles. It seems equally that the work of Costa ben Lucca—he described an inhaled spirit lodging in the heart[9] and revived Galen's idea of spirits moving through the ventricles, controlled by valves—were available in the East, and taken over by the Arabs.[10]

[5] Ibid., p. 100.
[6] K. D. Keele, op. cit., p. 56.
[7] L. J. Rather, *Mind and Body in Eighteenth-Century Medicine. A Study based on Jerome Gaub's 'De Regimine Mentis'*, London, 1965, p. 125.
[8] W. Pagel, op. cit., p. 103.
[9] M. D. Altschule, op. cit., p. 319.
[10] W. Pagel, op. cit., p. 101.

No theory becomes any more valid in its passage from one encyclopedia to another, and with the Arabs we find a strange mixture of basically Galenic ideas. With Haly Abbas[11] (tenth century) the brain is the seat of the reasonable soul, the origin of sense and voluntary motion. The front of the brain is soft, for perception and gives rise to sensory nerves. The back is correspondingly hard. The two front ventricles take in and expel air.

The ideas of Avicenna, in the next century, are more complex. Influenced by Aristotle, he described three souls in the body, physical (in the liver),[12] controlling digestion and evacuation, animal in the heart, responsible for appetite and anger, the fountainhead of the five senses, the source of imagination and movement, and the rational soul, not localized, exercising its faculties—thought and memory—in the brain. The heart, then, is the 'fountainhead' of the five senses: they are rooted here, *radicaliter*, but are exercised in the brain. They feed into the *sensus communis*, located in the forepart of the first ventricle, which has the capacity to judge between the senses and present its findings to the imagination. This, at the rear of the first ventricle, retains images from the *sensus communis* for the purposes of mental operation.[13] It will be noticed that these are functions of the animal (i.e. sentient) soul, although in the brain. The device of seating them *radicaliter* in the heart, but in practice in the brain, recalls that of the early Christian writers who had to reconcile the authorities putting the soul in the heart with those who placed it in the brain.

It will be noticed that while the neoplatonic-Christian soul as a single entity had had its faculties in the ventricles, the influence of Aristotle now suggested that these were faculties of the *sentient* (animal) soul. The influence of Plato encouraged the location of this in the heart and the vegetative in the liver. The absence of Christian influence enabled Avicenna to hold on to the concept that there were three distinct souls in the body.

These ideas were adopted almost completely by the West. Albertus Magnus, for example, takes Avicenna's views, and with other elements forges a coherent scheme of physiology and psychology. There is, he says at the beginning of *De Anima*,[14] only one soul, but he seems to forget this almost at once, and treats in the orthodox way of the vegetative, sensitive and rational souls. He is nevertheless quite explicitly dealing with the organs employed

11 P. de Koning, *Trois Traités d'Anatomie Arabes*, Leiden, 1903, p. 280.
12 A. J. Arberry, *Avicenna on Theology*, London, 1951, p. 50.
13 S. M. Afnan, *Avicenna. His Life and Works*, London, 1958, p. 138.
14 Albertus Magnus, *De Anima* (in *Philosophie Naturalis*, Venice, 1492).

by the faculties, and not the seats of the souls. There are five external and five internal senses. The external supply the *sensus communis* which distinguishes between them and enables its possessor to be conscious of perception. This is sited at the front of the first ventricle and feeds the imagination, at the back of this ventricle. The cogitative faculty in the middle ventricle rearranges the images derived from the imagination. The power of judgement is located at the top of this ventricle, and perceives the significance of this rearrangement. Lastly (unlike Avicenna) memory is placed in the posterior ventricle. All these, including memory, are powers of the *sensitive* soul; the intellect is 'an abstraction from matter' and does not have an organ in the body. Voluntary motion arises from the back of the brain, and involuntary from the heart, where also is the irascible virtue, and, unusually, the concupiscible.

Albertus' treatment of Avicenna was part of an increasing flow of Greek science in Arabian garb that was reaching the West during the thirteenth century. Aristotle's works became more widely known, as we may see in the Arabic-Latin translations of Alfred of Sarashel (the Englishman) or in Bartholomew of England's encyclopedia, where Aristotle's three souls are presented in addition to the ventricular theory. William of Saliceto, while locating the mental functions in the ventricles precisely as Albertus Magnus had done, nevertheless accepted that the heart was also sensitive.[15]

By the fourteenth century the influence of Aristotle threatened to eclipse the ventricular theory. Guy de Chauliac (who was also familiar with Galen's *De Usu Partium*) placed the *reasonable* soul in the brain, the faculties, previously of the sensitive soul, distributed in the ventricles in the usual way, but he regarded the heart as the instrument of all the virtues of body and soul, the paramount organ where the complete unity of body and soul is achieved.[16] To the ventricular theory Mondino[17] added the Aristotelian notion that the brain cooled the heart, and further, that intellect depended on an intact relationship of the heart and middle ventricle.

The battle continued into the fifteenth century. While an Aristotelian like Pico della Mirandola[18] made the heart the seat of vital force and the *sensorium commune*, we can point to Leonardo da Vinci[19] as a protagonist of the ventricular theory. Leonardo's early drawings of the ventricles are in the medieval tradition, but his

---

[15] William of Saliceto, *Cyrurgia*, Piacenza, 1476, cap. 'Anathomia' (unpaginated).
[16] *The Middle English Translation of Guy de Chauliac's Anatomy*, ed. Björn Wallner, Lund, 1964, p. 113.
[17] Mondino, *Anatomia*, ed. Dryander, Marburg, 1541, pp. 52, 56.
[18] W. Pagel, op. cit., p. 110.
[19] K. D. Keele, op. cit., p. 59.

masterly experiment of injecting them with wax led to much more accurate illustrations. Seeing that the cranial nerves seem to arise from the middle ventricle, he shifted the *sensorium commune* to here from the first ventricle. Attendant upon it was the soul. Later still he moved the sensory centre to the posterior ventricle because of its proximity to the spinal cord. As Leonardo's drawings are so accurate, it is best to drop the terminology of the ventricular theory. The 'first ventricle' in that hypothesis is of course double, so that the 'middle' ventricle corresponds to the modern third, and the posterior to the fourth. The spinal medulla was important to Leonardo, as he had found that a frog will live when deprived of all the organs normally thought to be seats of the soul: brain, heart and liver. We may recall the importance of this experiment to Whytt.

The ventricular theory finally disappeared during the first half of the sixteenth century. At the same time Aristotle's influence was receding before that of Galen, and the soul, in danger of returning to the heart, established itself in the substance of the brain. The change, however, had blurred some distinctions. The older writers had been careful to divorce the local appearance of the faculties from the localization of the soul itself, but now it was more easily assumed that the soul attended upon its faculties, and particularly upon the *sensus communis*, one of the functions of which, as we have seen, was to enable its owner to be aware of the process of perception: it was part of consciousness. Likewise these had been functions of the sensitive soul, but with the fusion of the lower souls into the upper, the distinction was lost.

In the meantime the ventricular theory carried on in a number of guises. In the rather medieval *Antropologium* of Magnus Hundt (1501), the brain is the seat of the *rational* soul, the faculties of which are distributed in the ventricles, and like Mondino, the brain is a cooling organ. The faculties are as usual except that the 'imaginative virtue', generally part of the cogitative faculty, is here imagination itself. The brain expands and contracts, and the movement of spirits through the ventricles which is associated with the mental operations, is controlled by various *anchae* which open and close the entrances to the ventricles. The heart is the organ of motion, the seat of the sensitive soul, and the formal origin of the veins, nerves, arteries and the faculties. The current debate on whether there are three souls is solved in the Aristotelian way by saying that the lower souls are contained in the highest as triangles within a square, and that the soul as the form of the body is *tota in toto et tota in qualibet parte totius*. These arguments are standard scholastic technique, and unremarkable, save that the *tota in toto* logic was often used to

113

show that in a real way the soul was coextensive with the body.[20] The books of Zerbis[21] and Reisch,[22] both of 1502, give the same account of the ventricles, Zerbis only adding that 'some say' the posterior part of the brain could be removed without loss of memory.

Jacopo Berangario da Carpi (1522)[23] removed all the faculties into the front ventricles, leaving the middle and posterior cavities to serve as conducting channels for spirits serving sense and motion. The 'red worm' (plexus choroides) controls mental operations. The heart, particularly its left ventricle, is the most noble organ, created first and the origin of the vital and critical heat.

Hundt's pictures of the ventricles appears, slightly altered, in Dryander's book on the anatomy of the body (1537)[24] probably by way of Laurenz Fries[25] (1518). The arrangement of the cranial nerves suggests it was constructed from Mondino's description (Dryander edited a version of Mondino) but in Dryander's explanation of the figure the functions of the ventricles are omitted. The text refers to the anterior *part* of the brain, which contains the power of cogitation and generates spirits which, flowing to the third ventricle, fulfil the duties of memory.

Perhaps this drift away from the ventricular theory was a humanist tendency, for Dryander was a pupil of Günther of Andernach. Certainly the increasing flow of translations direct from the Greek sources would have done little to perpetuate the theory. Perhaps the first influential refutation comes with Fernel's *De Naturali Parte Medicinae* of 1542. As has been suggested above, by now Galen's physiology had supplanted that of Aristotle, but the three souls of the latter are still the springs of action. Fernel remembers to say that the three are in fact faculties of a single soul, but like Albertus Magnus does not preserve this in his discussion. The *sensus communis*, memory and the 'constructive virtue' are still faculties of the sensitive soul, and are placed in the whole substance of the brain, not distinct from each other by seat.[26]

The remains of a Platonic system appear when Fernel includes the heart in the mechanism of ambition and anger, and the liver (and, with Galen, the mouth of the stomach) in that of appetite for food, but Fernel emphasizes that the true seat of these processes is the brain.

[20] M. Hundt, *Antroplogium*, Leipzig, 1501
[21] G. de Zerbis, *Liber Anathomie Corporis Humani*, Venice, 1502, p. 112.
[22] A. Crombie, *Augustine to Galileo*, London, Mercury Books, 1961, vol. 2, p. 196.
[23] J. Berengario da Carpi, *A Short Introduction to Anatomy (Isagoge Breves)*, (a translation by L. R. Lind of the 1523 ed.), Chicago, 1959, p. 143.
[24] Dryander, *Anatomiae, Hoc est, Corporis Humani Pars Prior*, Marburg, 1537.
[25] W. Pagel, op. cit., p. 114.
[26] J. Fernel, *De Naturali Parte Medicinae*, Paris, 1542, p. 89.

The ventricles themselves, 'inasfar as they are the receptacles of the spirits' are the instruments of sense and motion, in a Galenic way; likewise the harder substance at the posterior of the brain is more suited to motion: this part is the most likely seat of the sensitive soul. The fore-part of the brain is the *instrument* of sentience, while the special sense of touch is the care of the meningeal membranes. Mind is purely incorporeal and not related spatially to the body. The third soul, or faculty, the nutritive, is placed in the liver.

Pursuing the history of the ventricular theory, we have come a long way from Robert Whytt. It is not, however, without its significance. During the early period of the theory, the Aristotelian vegetative soul (and the sentient and rational insofar as they depended on it) as the form of the whole extent of the matter of a living organism, was often argued to be coextensive with it. Another argument for coextension was that the rational soul, being immaterial, must be related if to any then to all parts of the body. We have seen what similarity and historical connection this has to Whytt's ideas, by way of immateriality and the *tota in toto* argument. With the returning physiology of Galen, the faculties of the souls and often the souls themselves were distinct by seat in the body, and the *tota in toto* argument for coextension could no longer apply. The soul was now certainly whole in the whole body, but its parts were in the corresponding parts of the body: another kind of coextension, and more nearly related to Whytt's. Thus, for example, the powers of the nutritive soul, located in the liver, were nutrition, growth and reproduction. Growth was spread over the body, reproduction placed in the gonads and nutrition in the digestive organs. The latter was traditionally divided into the faculties of attraction, retention, digestion and expulsion, which were in turn to be found in the oesophagus, stomach, liver and intestines, organs suited to their functions. All organs thus fulfilled some duty of the soul, and the net result was the same as for other kinds of coextensive animism, whether Aristotle's or Whytt's. The soul by its presence not only enlivened each organ that it might fulfil the function of the soul to which it was best fitted, but gave direction to the activity toward the good of the whole.

By a devious piece of scholastic reasoning, even this Galenesque physiology could be reconciled to the *tota in toto* argument: the soul was potentially entire in all parts of the body, lacking expression only through want of organs; if the foot had an eye, it could see. We have seen how the coextensive soul of the ancient atomists was similar. The coextensive soul envisaged by Whytt was limited *to*, if not *by* the organs and tissues which contained it, but it is not unrelated to the souls of the ancient atomists and the medieval scholastics. One of the influences of the ventricular theory was to encourage devices of argument which could reconcile irrefutable but contradictory authorities. By envisaging potential presence, immaterial localization, *tota in toto* coextension and similar abstractions, the widely different views of Galen, Aristotle, Avicenna and the Church could be combined.

By Galen's influence, too, the nutritive faculties were contrasted to the vital faculties rather than to Aristotle's sentient soul, although both the latter had been seated in the heart. The sentient soul, it will be recalled, was responsible for most of the mental functions in the brain, the immaterial non-localized rational soul supplying only the higher form of reason, being an extrinsic 'accident' in scholastic terms. Perhaps the most direct result of the ventricular theory was to fix attention on the existence of a *sensus communis* in the brain. This faculty never really lost the connotation that it was *located*; by Whytt's time the term *sensorium commune* which can clearly mean 'the place where . . .' was in more common use, and, a fruit of the ventricular theory, was indispensable in considerations touching the soul, and reflex and sympathetic activity.

CHAPTER X

Whytt and the Soul

Leaving the ventricular theory behind, we return to those philosophers and physicians whose influence upon Whytt was direct. Their writings formed the basis of his education and an authoritative background from which he frequently quoted. Some of the changes made in the concept of the soul by the passage of the ventricular theory have been mentioned in the previous chapter; those which concern our consideration of Whytt were the arguments brought forward to prove coextension and the fixing of attention on the *sensus communis*. The most profound change, however, was that which contributed to Whytt's conception of the soul as single.

Just as in the earliest days of the ventricular theory most notice was taken, for religious reasons, of the highest of what were then the three Platonic souls, which thus had to accommodate the faculties of the lower. So one of the greatest changes between the end of the ventricular theory and Whytt (the other being the abolition of the soul by Descartes) was the assimilation by the extrinsic 'accident', the rational soul, of the properties of the two lower Aristotelian souls which disappeared, being already in the process of replacement by Galenic faculties.

All this took a great deal of time. Vesalius,[1] like Fernel rejecting the functions of the ventricles, nevertheless held that there were three souls. The principal of these was located in the brain and performed *all* the mental operations. This probably owes more to Plato than to an assimilation of the sentient soul by the rational, as the place of the former is taken by the 'irascible' soul, residing, said Vesalius, in the heart. The concupiscent soul was in the bowels.

The attribution of some of the powers traditionally associated with the sentient soul to the rational, one of those distinctions blurred, as we have noted, by the passage of the ventricular theory, led to the natural conclusion that animals, lacking rational souls, were mere machines. Periera (1544)[2] anticipated Descartes to this conclusion. That animals showed signs of memory and judgement

---

[1] C. Singer, *Vesalius on the Human Brain*, London, 1952, p. 1.
[2] L. D. Cohen, 'Descartes and Henry More on the beast-machine', *Ann. Sci.*, 1936, *1*, 48.

was of course a reason why all these mental faculties except reason had in the strict Aristotelian tradition been assigned to the sentient soul, the rational soul supplying the uniquely human kind of reason. Whytt rejected the Cartesian animals as mere pieces of clockwork and approached the Aristotelian position in allowing that the mental functions of animals proceeded from their sentient principles, which differed from the human soul in degree rather than kind. Rather than attribute sentient souls to animals and rational souls to men, Whytt preferred to imagine a scale terminating in man, along which were stationed animals in relation to the extent of their intelligence. This variation among the orders of creation was imposed upon the soul by the exigencies of singularity. Whytt's soul, single for religious reasons, inherited by assimilation the different modes of existence of the old triple-hierarchy of souls.

The first stage in this assimilation of the lower souls into the upper was the fusion of the two lower souls themselves: they were more like each other than either was like the rational soul. This could be expressed in scholastic terms as in Biondo's *De Anima Dialogus* of 1545;[3] the vegetative and sentient souls were both 'forms' of matter, and in animals constituted together a 'mixed form'. Man also had an 'animated' form, the highest immaterial Aristotelian soul. His soul was therefore double. In a different way, Biondo's authority, St. Augustine, had compressed the three Platonic souls into one: Biondo's was a deliberate attempt to reduce the tripartite Aristotelian soul to one for the demands of theology. Another point of interest is that this *tota in toto* coextensive soul was bound by no law to the body but was free to act as it chose. This was the major point of the Stahlian doctrine, and Whytt vigorously opposed it.

Theologians might be expected to go further. The theological compendium of De Combis (1554)[4] scarcely mentions the Aristotelian division of the soul, which is a non-dimensional unity placed, however, in the heart. De Combis is well informed on medical matters, and his problem is to reconcile the Aristotelian heart with the Galenesque brain. This he does by resorting to a device already mentioned: the soul is *radicaliter* in the heart, and uses the brain as an instrument. The *sensus communis* is the principal of the internal senses, and is seated in that place 'where the five sensitive nerves come together, which is medullary and humid'.[5] The usual other internal senses are distributed in the substance of the brain from back to front, except fantasy, which is in 'the middle

[3] Biondo, *De Anima Dialogus*, Rome, 1545
[4] I. de Combis, *Compendium Totium Theologicae Veritatis*, Venice, 1554.
[5] Ibid., p. 78.

118

of the middle cellule'. This looks like a reversion to the ventricular theory, but we should not be too critical of De Combis, for the noted anatomist Colombo[6] even later insisted that memory lay in the fourth ventricle.

The philosophers were not in such a hurry to rid themselves of the three souls of Aristotle, and we may again see an intermediate stage in a discussion about souls as conceived by the peripatetics written by Petrus Duodus in 1575.[7] The faculties of the soul(s) in man may be measured in scholastic terms of 'intension' and 'latitude'. By juggling with 'grades of latitudes' etc., and the 'triangle within a square' argument, Duodus shows that whether the soul be single or multiple, all its faculties are in every part. The difficulty of stretching the argument to cover all three souls was really, however, still unsurmountable, and Duodus settles for uniting the two lower grades of soul as they both depend on matter, and contrasting the result with the purely immaterial and non-dimensional higher soul. Again, as in Biondo, man has a double soul.

Duodus was aware of the experiment of dividing insects, and allowed that both halves contained a part of the soul (naturally, the lower of the two). Thus the lower soul was coextensive with the body, and further, was typical of the matter it occupied; of all parts, the heart was the most important.

Again, physicians looked at the matter from an angle slightly different from that of the theologians and philosophers, and Cesalpino and Zabarella[8] may be mentioned as adherents to the belief that there were three souls or faculties in the Aristotelian way, and that the brain was merely the sensitive instrument of the soul rooted in the heart. This soon led to change of some significance. It could no longer be denied that the nerves were the agents of sense and motion, and it seemed reasonable that the *sensorium* was at their common termination. Many agreed with Piccolhomineus[9] (1586) in placing the soul at this *sensorium*.

A full and scholarly discussion is found in the *Problema* of Nicolas Nancel[10]: *An sedes animae in cerebro? An in corde? aut ubi denique?* (1582). He examines the historical material, including that which we have already met in Soranus and Tertullian, and wisely decides that the different opinions of the seat of the soul in the Hippocratic

[6] W. Pagel, op. cit., p. 102.

[7] P. Duodus, *Peripeticarum de Anima*, Venice, 1575.

[8] W. Pagel, op. cit., p. 106.

[9] A. Piccolhomineus, *Anatomicae Praelectiones*, Rome, 1582, pp. 265-9.

[10] N. Nancel, *Problema, An Sedes Animae in Corde? An in Cerebro, aut ubi Denique est?* (1582), in *De Immortalitate Animae*, Paris, 1587.

collection is due to their different authorship. He accepts completely that the soul is single, and places it in the brain at the termination of the nerves. The compromise is now shifting to the Galen end of the scale: the faculties of the soul, says Nancel, although exercised in different organs (nutrition in the liver, anger etc. in the heart) are all rooted with the soul in the brain. He is reversing the device by which others had explained Galen on the basis of Aristotle. Nancel follows Galen on the generation of the animal spirit, the servant of the soul, and is impressed with the evidence that many animals survive the loss of their hearts for a brief period; clearly these cannot be seats of the soul.

In discussing the opinion of an ancient authority (which he claims as his own) that the mind seems to move from the brain to the heart in certain states of thought, Nancel argues that mind is an immaterial faculty of the soul and, unrelated to matter, is 'tota in toto . . .', although he prefers to say it is diffused through the body. It is interesting to note that he uses the same scholastic argument that Whytt quoted in support of his idea of the coextensive yet indivisible soul, the mind was like God, who, as immortal, was immaterial, as matter was subject to decay, and as immaterial was not subject to place: He was in every *ubi*, but not in any place.

Similar arguments are found in Laurens' book on the sense of vision, written in 1599: the soul is single, indivisible and wholly in all parts, yet principally seated in the brain. Its principal lower forces, anger and nutrition, no longer occupy the heart and liver even in Nancel's limited sense. The faculties simply appear in the organs fulfilling these functions. The previous distinction between the sentient and rational souls has been lost: the imagination, previously an attribute of the sentient soul, takes on some appearance of reason, and the soul of animals is less complete than the old sentient soul. On the question of the function of the ventricles, Laurens concludes that the opinion of the Arabs was specious but vulgarly accepted, while the Greeks (by putting the faculties in the substance of the brain) 'had plaid the more subtile Philosophers'.[11]

The *Opera Omnia* of the elder Riolan[12] (1610) contain much that is more old-fashioned than the date suggests. The sentient soul is responsible for the traditional mental faculties, and imagination remains in the anterior ventricle. Like others before him, Riolan says that the soul is single and *tota in toto* . . . as the form of the animal, but treats of each Aristotelian soul as separately as Albertus

[11] A. Laurens, *A Discourse on the Preservation of the Sight; of Melancholike Diseases; and of Old Age*, trans. R. Surphlet, London, 1599, p. 80.
[12] J. Riolan, *Opera Omnia*, Paris, 1610, pp. 48, 60.

120

Magnus had done. In this way the rational soul is the *animus*, and both vegetal and sentient souls are *anima*, the usual distinction in terminology which aided the fusion of the vegetal and sentient souls into one.

Riolan was aware that excised portions of insects survive longer than those of more perfect animals, and attributed this to the continued activity of a soul: the soul, being entirely in the whole *and* the parts, was potentially present with all its faculties even in the excised portion, but was prevented from manifesting these powers by the absence of the necessary organs. The rational soul was similarly coextensive and only prohibited from cogitation in distant or separated organs by the absence of the *phantasmata*, its essential organs in the brain.

Although it was, as usual, the sentient soul which performed the mental functions (except reason) Riolan speaks of the *animus* seeing through the eye, and, particularly, knowing itself to see by virtue of the *sensus communis*. This association of the soul and the *sensus communis* became more important when the soul was thought to be single: the common sense was either the seat of or the last material link to the soul.

As the essential organs of the rational soul were the *phantasmata* so the essential organs of the sentient soul were the nerves, so although coextensive, it could not feel in parts destitute of nerves, and its effective seat was therefore the brain. The necessary organs of the vegetative soul were the liver and heart. This limitation of the powers of the soul to the proper tissues recalls Whytt's idea, and we may assume that Whytt, who quoted from Riolan on the subject of sensitivity in sympathy, had a wider acquaintance with the latter's works.

A determined attempt to restore the Aristotelian concept of the soul was made in 1616 by Fortuni Liceti, who wrote and published in the Aristotelian university of Padua *De Animarum Coextensione Corpore*. His argument is founded upon the necessary dependence of the rational and sentient souls upon the vegetative, which was most easily shown to be coextensive with the body. As all parts of the body are nourished, so must the vegetative or nutritive soul be present at those parts as the primary efficient cause, for, as Aristotle said, all action is by contact. Growth likewise occurs in all parts and in plants at least the other function of the vegetative soul, reproduction, is possessed by most parts. Again, the persistence of life in an excised part indicates the presence of soul. Lastly, vital heat extends all over the body.

The sentient soul is spatially identifiable with the vegetative not only because it depends on vital heat (the action of which must be by contact) but also because its own functions are spread through the body. The sense of touch is universal and the special senses potentially so: if eyes were present in the feet then these extremities would see. The soul, that is to say, is limited in function by the absence of functional organs, an idea originating with the Greek atomists and turning up in a variety of authors (like Riolan) until Whytt's elaboration of it.

Liceti begins to depart more seriously from contemporary opinions when he suggests that the *sensus communis* is coextensive with the body. The association of this and the soul, seen in Riolan, is emphasized: it is 'either the substance of the soul itself or is inseparable from it',[13] but here it is strictly the sentient soul forming the association. The argument centres around the extent of sensation in the body. In a similar way, *phantasia*, as a cause of local motion, is distributed over the entire body; the nerves cannot act as instruments of a centralized soul, but the soul must be at the site of their activity, as the form acting by contact. The sentient soul animates all organs (it sees in the eyes, and hears in the ears, etc.) with the exception of bone and cartilage, and is divisible on the division of the body.

Lastly, the rational soul, God-given and immaterial, has no need of a spatial relation to matter; nevertheless, its power to govern the activities of the sentient soul and the body argue strongly to Liceti that it is coextensive. If it were not, the part to which it did not reach would be merely animal or even plant, and could not be human. The intellect, or rational soul is the Substantial Form of the body and must be coextensive. Although the argument derives from Aristotle, Liceti remarks on the 'absurdity' of Aristotle in placing the soul in the heart. In arriving at a *tota in toto . . .* coextension, Liceti uses, like Whytt, the argument that God is everywhere in the universe.

The dispute between the Aristotelians and Galenists continued. In the mid-seventeenth century Caspar Hofmann collected and published a series of papers[14] putting forward both views, many of which had been published in the early part of the century. Thus Julius Caesar Claudinus,[15] following Galen, placed the faculties of the soul in the substance of the brain, while Ludovic Buccaferrea held the Aristotelian tenet that the mind was seated in the heart, to which he added that it acted in the brain, a com_promise we have met before. As a compromise, this device was

---

[13] F. Liceti, *De Animarum Coextensione Corpore*, Padua, 1616, p. 25.

[14] C. Hofmann, *Pro Veritate Opellae tres*, Paris, 1647.

[15] J. C. Claudinus, *Quaestio, an Facultates Principes Animae secundum Sedes Distinguantur in Cerebro?*, 1617.

122

elaborated by Sennert[16] and others, who said not only was the soul rooted in the heart and manifest only secondarily in the brain, but also that nerves and blood vessels, the servants of the soul, had their immaterial but true origins in the heart, performing their functions as physical entities from the brain and liver.

This dispute never recovered from the blow dealt it by Harvey. In 1616, when the Paduan Liceti published his book, Harvey, who had studied at Padua and was equally Aristotelian, was already lecturing on the circulation of the blood. The full exposition was published in 1628. Its first effect was to demolish the liver as a seat of the soul. The scheme of physiology derived from Galen had held that the nutritive soul, or faculty, was located here and its operations dispensed to all parts of the body by way of the veins. Now that the veins had finally been shown to spring from the heart, the liver was displaced from its central position. (We have seen how this had already happened in the case of Laurens, with whose textbook Harvey was familiar, and who had said all veins arise from the heart.) The liver died as the seat of a soul, and Bartholin wrote its epitaph.

The heart fared little better. Although it was a restoration of an Aristotelian idea to attribute the origin of the veins to the heart, the Aristotelian idea of the heart as the seat of the soul suffered with the acceptance of that organ as a muscular pump. Harvey himself was at first uncertain on the question of the seat of the soul. At all events, the heart retained for him a non-conscious sensibility, which was not referred to the *sensorium* in the brain. From it arose involuntary motions. This sensibility resembles Whytt's 'simple sensation', the non-conscious feeling of separated muscles or lowly animals like oysters. Like Whytt's, too, it was responsible for the continued activity of (an example they both quoted) a decapitated fowl.

In his manuscript notes on the local motion of animals (1627)[17] Harvey shows a mixture of ideas on the soul. Sometimes he speaks of the blood as containing the soul, which corresponds to the fiery element of the stars. This recalls the 'perfection' that the blood undergoes in the heart, and may lie behind his brief reference to Robert Fludd, who not only held that the body contained three rather Aristotelian souls (the rational in the head) but also a *pneuma*, celestial, the origin of wisdom, breathed into the blood and heart. Servet,[18] who was concerned in the discovery of the

[16] D. Sennert, *Opera*, Paris, 1641, vol. 1, p. 83.
[17] W. Harvey, *De Motu Locali Animalium*, notes of 1627, ed. and trans. by G. Whitteridge, Cambridge, 1959.
[18] S. Toulmin and J. Goodfield, op. cit., p. 350.

pulmonary circulation, also held that the soul was a kind of *pneuma* taken in by the mouth and seated in the blood.

As a cause of animal motion, Harvey recognizes kinds or divisions of soul. Just as the power of simple sentience could be shown to reside in the heart of a fowl by decapitation, so is the 'sensitive and motive soul' in the brain of a frog which moves after its heart is removed. Is then the brain the prime mover?, asks Harvey in the notes. The commander? The architect? Or rather (and this seems nearer to his own inclinations) is the heart the ruler?

By the time he wrote *De Generatione Animalium*, Harvey seems to have made up his mind. The soul, he says[19] unequivocally, is in the blood. Ontogenetically the first-born and the first-bearing, the blood is the primary organ of the body, possessing those characteristics that Aristotle had attributed to the heart. Alive *per se*, it was animated: it was the sole vehicle of the soul and the carrier of the soul's immediate agents, spirit and innate heat. Again the soul corresponds to the substance of the stars, and is 'the vicar of omnipotent God'. The blood has thus a double nature. 'Materially' it is partly nutriment for the organs it visits, and 'formally' considered it is endued with heat and spirit, the agents of its most important constituent the soul, which, carried to all parts, is coextensive with the body.

In this chapter on the blood, Harvey is concerned with refuting the common idea that the blood served only as a food, and particularly the conception that venous and arterial blood had different nutritional functions. Although still speaking of 'coctions', he points out that the circulation of the blood prohibited any distinction of function, that the liver, in other words, no longer the origin of the veins, could not be a special digestive organ in the old sense—the seat of the nutritive soul.

In this chapter, too, is Harvey's account of how he (and the King) were able to touch the heart of the eldest son of the viscount of Montgomery, which was exposed as the result of an accident. This is the story Whytt refers to in his dispute with Haller over the sensibility of the heart and we may assume that Whytt was familiar with the rest of Harvey's account of the blood, including the coextensive soul (and its clear relationship to earlier ideas). Although, said Harvey, the blood is the first-born organ and the seat of the soul, it does not itself offer evidence of sensibility and irritability. This is manifest in the *punctum saliens*, the heart at its first embryological appearance. Whytt[20] also quotes this passage to show that

[19] W. Harvey, *Exercitationes de Generatione Animalium*, London, 1651, p. 154.
[20] *Works*, p. 298.

irritability is proportional to sensibility, and we have already seen (p.82) how he took as a starting point for his explanation of the motion of the heart Harvey's account of how the blood stimulates the *punctum saliens* into motion.

The effect of Harvey's discovery on his contemporaries seems to have discouraged speculation on the seat and nature of the lower soul or souls. If the vegetative soul had no seat, did it exist? Attention was again concentrated on the rational soul and the sensitive soul, both seated in the brain. While in the previous century the vegetative and sentient souls were inclined to be grouped together as they both depended on matter, now that they no longer had distinct seats, the fusion was complete, and the result was a new *anima*.

While the sentient soul had been absorbed by the vegetative, as they were both 'forms' of matter (as in Biondo and Duodus) its faculties, taken to the head by the ventricular theory, became confused with the rational soul, and were assimilated by it. This joint product was the *animus*, the immortal immaterial reasoning gift of God. Thus Gassendi[21] postulated an *anima* which was material and passed on from one generation to another, like that described by Tertullian and Epicurus, with whom he was not unacquainted. To this was added the divine *animus*, introduced into the foetus some time after conception. These points were embodied in a letter to Thomas Fyens (1629) who expressed a belief that the rational soul reached the foetus on the third day (1620).[22]

Whytt pointed out that the arguments used to favour an extended soul could also be employed in support of a coextensive soul, and he relied partly upon Gassendi as an authority for the former proposition. No one in Gassendi's time would deny that an *anima* such as his was material and as a consequence extended; the point at issue concerned the *animus* (Whytt uses 'soul' and gives no suggestion of Gassendi's *anima* and *animus*) and did not arise until after Descartes, when we shall meet Gassendi again. At all events, this *anima* of Gassendi was composed of atoms of a nature similar to fire, diffused throughout the body, producing vital heat (principally in the right ventricle of the heart) and responsible for nutrition and movement. The similarity to the Greek atomists is marked, and it is not surprising that Whytt drew on both.

Gassendi added, in a closer parallel to Whytt, that the *anima* was responsible for the sentience of which both halves of a divided insect are clearly capable, and in the same way it felt pain locally

[21] G. S. Brett, *The Philosophy of Gassendi*, London, 1908, p. 108.
[22] R. Watt, *Bibliotheca Britannica*, Edinburgh, 1827, vol. I, p. 367.

in the body if the nervous connection of that part to the brain were intact.[23] This is very similar to Whytt's statement that a muscle (for instance) is sensitive in and out of the body by the local action of the soul.

The new philosophy was as mechanical for others as it was corpuscular for Gassendi. Hobbes'[24] ideas on the mechanism of sensation which later illustrated this tendency are anticipated by some notes he made in about 1630, which suggest a physical chain of events between the sense organ and brain.

The effect of the doctrines of Descartes, the arch-mechanist, on ideas of the soul was revolutionary. He abolished the sentient-cum-vegetative soul and of its functions relegated the external senses and reflected motions of the sentient and all the faculties of the vegetative part to the mechanism of the body, elevating the internal senses to the rational soul. This hastened the process of the disappearance of the *anima*, but the completion of the process was achieved by the assimilation of the *anima* into the *animus* rather than by the exercise of what might be called René Descartes' razor.

Descartes put the soul into the pineal gland. This organ seemed suitable as it was single and conveniently placed in the midst of the spirits. Besides, it was being discussed as a seat of the soul at the time. (*L'Homme* was completed in 1633 but published posthumously in 1662. Much of his system was published in *Discours de la Méthode* of 1637). The quite immaterial soul was a 'thinking substance' and the body, including the spirits of the brain and nerves, was an 'extended substance' and obeyed purely physical laws. We need not be concerned with Descartes' physiology or mechanism of sensation, as it is well known and outside our subject, but one point should be noticed: Descartes said that in voluntary motion, the soul moved the pineal gland and altered the flow of spirits. In doing so he pinpointed a problem which had always lurked in the background of body-soul relationships: how could a purely immaterial soul affect the matter of the body? The old quasi-material soul, or the spirits had effected this, but they were not available to Descartes, *ex hypothesi*. Further, the soul, being immaterial, was unextended. Gassendi thought that 'interaction' of body and soul as Descartes described it was impossible. How could the soul (apart from its immateriality) act simultaneously at the termination of several nerves, if it were unextended? The *animus* must be extended in the brain. Whytt[25] quoted Gassendi in showing that as nerves are physical structures with finite and irreducible diameters,

[23] K. D. Keele, op. cit., p. 76.
[24] T. Hobbes, *The Elements of Law*, ed. F. Tonnies, Cambridge, 1928, p. 152.
[25] *Works*, p. 201.

126

their common termination must be extended, and so the soul whether or not immaterial, must also be at least coextensive with this *sensorium*.

The 'occasionalism' of Malebranche[26] avoided the difficulties of inter-action in another way, and the 'pre-established harmony' of Liebnitz[27] escaped the problem altogether at the cost of a rather elaborate philosophical scheme, which denied a causal relationship between soul and body; Whytt said it was 'an ingenious fable'. Another way out was that espoused by Spinoza, who had argued against Descartes that the nerves do not extend to the ventricles, that the location of the pineal is unsuited to movement, and, primarily, that interaction between the material and immaterial was impossible. His answer to this *impasse* was to assume a strict unity of existence, so that 'body' and 'soul' were not separate entities. Thus his definition of God includes material extension, and his concept of mind is inseparable from that of body.[28]

It has already been noted that one of the influences of Descartes was to hasten the disappearance of a multiple soul; the other was to make credible certain physiological actions into which the soul did not enter at all. Previously all bodily actions had been thought as a matter of course to be governed by the soul, whether it was extended to these parts of the body or not, but now that the soul was curtailed in function, it became easier to imagine it limited also to one organ of the body. Neither idea was, of course, admissible to Whytt, as we have seen. For him, Descartes' soulless animals were 'so many curious pieces of clockwork wound up and set agoing'.[29] Otherwise, the details of the Cartesian scheme did not long survive. The pineal was shown to be unsuitable by the absence of sufficient blood vessels and nerves, and the frequent presence of calcification or disease. Many replaced it with other cerebral organs, and some, like Sir Thomas Browne, could find no organ in the body for the rational soul.[30] There was a general reaction against Descartes, but it did not destroy the usefulness of the analogy he had drawn, and mechanistic physiology pursued its course into the next century.

This reaction took a variety of forms. Henry More was not

[26] A. Crombie, op. cit., vol. 2, p. 313.
[27] See for example, R. L. Shaw, *Leibniz*, Penguin Books, 1954, p. 143. Leibniz made it even clearer than before that Cartesian interaction was impossible. See L. J. Rather, 'G. E. Stahl's Psychological Physiology', p. 45, footnote.
[28] H. A. Wolfson, *The Philosophy of Spinoza*, New York, 1958, book 1, p. 80, book 2, pp. 48, 62, 337.
[29] *Works*, p. 153. For the later history of this phrase see chapter 12.
[30] D. Guthrie, *A History of Medicine*, 1958, p. 212.

opposed entirely to Descartes, and exchanged a series of letters[31] with him on the subject of the soulless state of brutes. He was, however, much influenced by neoplatonism, and insisted that the soul was extended. Whytt speaks of him as one of the greatest philosophers of the seventeenth and eighteenth centuries to argue for the extension of the soul. The others were Gassendi, Newton and Samuel Clarke.[32] Other authors, like Back (1648)[33] held the rare but recurring idea that the meninges were the *sensorium commune* (increasingly associated with the soul), on the basis of their softness and apparant connection with the coats of the nerves. The persistence of older ideas can still be seen, for example in Ecchard Leichner (1650)[34] for whom the soul is now quite single, possessed (by assimilation) of the lower faculties and is entirely in the whole body, and wholly in all its parts.

Perhaps the greatest rejection of Descartes was what might be called the animist reaction, in which we must include Whytt. This had its origins among the iatro-chemists, and had centred round an *archeus* which was identifiable with or similar to the soul. The *archeus* was introduced by Basil Valentine in the fifteenth century, and taken up by Paracelsus in the sixteenth. For him, *archei* in the organs governed the physiological processes, yet he speaks of a soul in the heart,[35] which used the brain as an instrument of reason. Van Helmont was a pre-Cartesian (his work was published only after his death in 1644) whose name is associated with the development of this idea. The sensitive soul he placed at the pyloric opening of the stomach, the movements and digestive processes of which it controlled. The stomach and spleen with the principle *archeus*, mortal but immaterial, acted, necessarily, together, upon a hierarchical system of inferior agencies, each devoted to an organ or function.

The stomach was chosen by Van Helmont because of its association with digestion, the six processes of which ultimately (at the fifth stage) produced the vital spirit of the *archeus* from the arterial blood, and then (the sixth stage) the *archeus* enabled the body to assimilate its nourishment. The similarities to Aristotle and Galen are clear. Secondly, the stomach had strong connections, nervous and in some way sympathetic with the brain, the organ and

[31] L. D. Cohen, op. cit.

[32] *Works*, p. 202.

[33] From J. D. Gohl, *Insufficientia Cerebri ad Sensum et Motum Expenditur*, Amsterdam, 1712, p. 48.

[34] E. Leichner, *De Invisibili et Totali Cujusque Animae in toto suo Corpore et Singulis ejus Partibus*, Erfurt, 1650.

[35] W. Pagel, op. cit., p. 107.

instrument of sense and motion. The meninges seem to have been of some importance. Van Helmont swallowed aconite and 'felt himself thinking in the stomach';[36] this power of thinking and indeed consciousness would be lost if the soul were damaged by a blow in the stomach.

The soul, controlling all bodily events, began its own diseases as a measure to safeguard the body by emitting dangerous matter, by sending 'acid ferments, or juices to various parts of the body'. (This later became a point of the Stahlian doctrine.) This sensitive soul was possessed by man alone.

Owing something to Van Helmont and Paracelsus, and to some extent anticipating Stahl, was the later animism of Claudius Perrault. This shows an interesting stage in the evolution of the old divided soul into eighteenth-century unitary animism. His physiology assumed two levels of consciousness, acute for dealing with external objects, corresponding to the old *animus*, and a lower consciousness to respond to otherwise imperceptible internal changes, as did the *anima* or sentient soul. He appears to have held that sensation was localized throughout the nerves, and thus coextensive with the body.

Stahl and his followers must be reckoned as the most important contributors to this animist reaction to Descartes. Their beliefs and relationship to Whytt are discussed below.

Apart from this animist reaction, the most important figure in the history of the soul between Descartes and Whytt was Thomas Willis, Sidleian Professor of Natural Philosophy at Oxford, who was something of a mechanist. He was, however, far from accepting Cartesian doctrines, particularly in relation to the soul. In the *Cerebri Anatome*,[37] Willis argued that the conarium, or pineal body, could not be the seat of the soul, as the Cartesians held, since it was possessed by other animals which did not show higher mental faculties.

Willis believed that imagination was seated in the *corpus callosum*. The soul (the 'lucid', the higher of the two souls) itself, of which imagination was a function, was diffused, 'radiant and beamy' through the whole head and its 'nervous dependencies' and the animal spirits were its fountain. The imagination was conscious perception, and was behind the *sensorium commune* (in the *corpus striatum*) in the sequence of perception. Only if an impression reached the *corpus callosum* from the 'common sensory' did a conscious sensation arise: perception involved contraction of the soul, motion its expansion.

---

[36] J. R. Partington, 'Joan Baptista van Helmont'. *Ann. Sci.*, 1936, *1*, 359.
[37] London, 1664.

Willis placed the seat of the imagination here because of the position of the callous bodies: he considered the nerves to end in the 'streaky or chamfered' bodies, the *corpora striata*. These streaks, he claimed, were aligned up and down, to and from the seat of perception or imagination, and were subservient to sense, and to motion. The streaks, then, were to be considered analogous if not continuous with the nerves, the terminations of which bounded the chamfered bodies upon one side, while the callous bodies were located upon the other. A sensation was capable of being 'reflected' back from the streaky bodies to initiate motion without stimulating consciousness. The importance of this in the history of the reflex allies Willis to Whytt, who similarly thought that a motion could be unconsciously reflected by part of the soul in the brain, or more importantly, by that in the spinal cord.

A similar 'reflection', said Willis, took place from the centre of consciousness: 'But if this sensible impression reaches the *callous body* (having passed the common sensory) stirs up the imagination, and the Spirits, reflecting from there and flowing back toward the Nervous Appendix, raise up the Appetite and local motions . . .'.[38]

Thus the mechanism of perception was a sequence of events which Willis located in a sequence of anatomical structures. Memory he placed in the cortex of the brain, and described the process of perception and memory thus:

That as often as the exterior part of the soul being struck, a sensible impression, as it were of the Optic Species, or as an undulation or waving of waters, is carried more inward, bending toward the chamfered bodies, a perception or inward sense of sensation outwardly had or received, arises. If that impression, being carried further, passes through the *callous body*, imagination follows the sense: Then if the same fluctuation of Spirits is struck against the *cortex* of the brain, as its utmost banks, it impresses on it the images or character of the sensible object, which when it is afterward reflected or bent back, raises up the memory of the same thing.[39]

The 'exterior part of the soul' was that at the extremities of the nerves, perceiving the 'sensibilium species'[40] and by its undulations or emanations an impulse was carried along the nerves to the seat of sensation. The animal spirits were the agents of this process, in the pores of the brain. The spirits were delivered from both cerebrum and cerebellum and filled the 'oblong marrow'. This Willis traced to its bifurcation and double termination at the

[38] T. Willis, *The Anatomy of the Brain*, p. 96. From *The Remaining Medical Works*.
[39] Ibid., p. 95.
[40] T. Willis, *De Anima Brutorum*, London, 1672, p. 107.

corpora striata: its function was to carry sensory and motor impressions to the correct nerves. Willis confirmed his ideas from post-mortem examinations of the brains of persons who had suffered a palsy. He found several with atrophied *corpora striata*.

Willis retained the old idea that the soul was divided into a higher and lower; the higher was the self-conscious intellectual soul of man; the lower, common to men and animals, itself consisted of parts, the vital and sensitive. Like that of the older philosophers, the vital soul was 'flamy' and was enkindled in the blood: it depended on the state of the body in a similar way to a flame which needs air and fuel. Willis seems to owe something to Bacon, for whom vital spirits were a breath of flame and air—the sort of surviving *pneuma* idea expressed by Fludd—while the inspiration from the atomism of Gassendi cannot be ignored.

Both parts of the soul were spatially distinct from each other: the lucid soul had its seat in the brain and 'its Appendix'—the nerve cord—which the 'flamy' soul was unable to enter, its seat being the blood. It consisted 'in the motion and agglomeration or heaping together of the most subtile and agil particles'.[41] This part of the soul, like Whytt's single soul, later, and many earlier souls, was coextensive with body: 'The corporeal soul, common to the more perfect brutes and man, is extended to the whole organic body'.[42] Its extension to the muscles, however, was not a cause of their contraction, as it was for Whytt. Willis held that muscle contraction was due to explosions of spirits arriving at and dilating the muscles; he mentioned that some believed contraction was due to the activity of the soul in the muscle, but dismisses the idea as involving what would be a corporeal soul with a supernatural agency. Thus Willis' corporeal soul represented the *anima*[43] and the lucid soul the *animus*, possessed by assimilation of many of the functions of the old sentient soul.

Willis' doctrines were criticized by, among others, Walter Charleton[44] who nevertheless himself envisaged a separate *anima* which vivified the body in the orthodox way[45] while the rational soul inhabited the grey matter of the brain.[46]

[41] T. Willis, *The Anatomy of the Brain*, p. 33.

[42] T. Willis, *De Anima Brutorum*, p. 38.

[43] W. Battie, *A Treatise on Madness*, London, 1758, p. 32, describes Willis as 'inventing' the anima and Stahl as deifying it.

[44] A. Meyer and R. Hierons, 'On Thomas Willis's concept of neurophysiology', *Med. Hist.*, 1965, *9*, 1, 142.

[45] W. Pagel, 'The reaction to Aristotle in seventeenth-century biological thought', *Science, Medicine and History, Essays in Honour of Charles Singer*, ed. E. A. Underwood, Oxford, 1953, vol. I, p. 497.

[46] R. Hunter and I. MacAlpine, *Three Hundred Years of Psychiatry*, London, 1966, p. 193.

After Willis various other structures within the brain were put forward as seats of the soul until the eighteenth-century reaction against this sort of speculation. At the same time the idea of a separate *anima* dropped out of use, and the single soul assumed its duties. Thus Honoratus Faber (1666)[47] includes the lower souls not very convincingly in the higher, as had often been done before, and places it, centralized, in the choroid plexus. Nicholaus Hoboken,[48] on the other hand, deals with a soul which is perfectly single, being both *anima* and *mens*. In *De Sede Animae* (1669) he says the sensorium is stretched along the medulla of the brain and cerebellum, at the origin of all the nerves. The cerebellum was responsible for simple and spontaneous sensations and motions, and the soul was most closely associated with that part of the *sensorium* in the brain. As almost everyone since Galen had said, the brain was suited to this office by its softness, dampness, coldness and abundance of spirits. The spirits were prepared in this medulla of the brain, and if one had to delve further for a more precise location of the soul then it would lie deeper, in a specific *meditullium*. Memory was to be found in those protuberances called the *nates* and *testes*. The brain in general was the primary seat of the soul, the *quasi-curia regalis*, and the cerebellum the secondary seat, the *quasi-vicaria curia*. In the latter the soul, like that of Whytt and Willis, acted unconsciously in producing spontaneous motions.

Another author we may note in the post-Willis-Descartes period is Diricus Dreyer,[49] whose tract on the soul (1677) locates the *anima* [*sic*] *rationalis* in the pineal, but allows it complete dominance of the body, 'reaching all parts by its operations'.[50] In this way he solved the *tota in toto* question. In other respects it corresponds to Descartes' *anima*; Dreyer puts emphasis on the generation of spirits by the 'choroid and retiform plexuses'. Dreyer was impressed, possibly more than we should be, by the reasoning of Dr. Tobias Andreae, who was assured by his own cogitations that man could conceive all his organs in his imagination clearly, if somewhat remotely, as if in a mirror, with the sole exception of the pineal gland, which defied the most earnest introspection; he drew an analogy with the eye which as the terminus of vision could perceive all organs but itself.

Other writers who made some kind of compromise between the

[47] H. Faber, *Tractatus Duo*, (2, *De Homine*) Paris, 1666, bk. 6, pp. 63, 67.
[48] N. Hoboken, *De Sede Animae seu Mentis Humani*, Utrecht, 1669, pp. 283, 283, 284, 290.
[49] D. Dreyer, *Specimen Tractationis Physicae de Sede aut potius Modo Praesentialitatis Animae Rationalis in Corpore Hominis*, Bremen, 1677.
[50] Ibid., p. 5.

views of Descartes and Willis were D. Duncan (1678)[51] who explained animal motions with a Cartesian mechanism yet from faculties of the soul distributed in the brain in a Willisian manner, and G. B. de Saint Romain,[52] an atomist for whom the soul was in the pineal, perception and common-sense in the ventricles, imagination and judgement in the *corpus callosum* and memory in the 'ashy substance'. Probably no one ever achieved greater variety for the seat of the soul than this!

R. de Vieussens, whose *Neurographia Universalis* was a textbook of some importance, was essentially a follower of Willis. Both put the *sensorium commune* in the *corpora striata*, but Vieussens thought that imagination was located in the *centrum ovale*, where also spirits were separated from the blood. The two structures were the origin of the nerves, and Vieussens grouped *both* as a *sensus communis*; this probably reflects the confusion which had always existed in some quarters between the imagination and the *sensus communis*, and certainly indicated that Vieussens thought of the *sensorium* as a place (the origin of the nerves) and the *sensus communis* as a faculty.[53] By Whytt's time the term sensorium had become general, and he himself always used it to suggest the place at the termination of the nerves where the soul exercised its most complex unconscious, and its conscious activities. In this he agreed with Willis and Vieussens. He disagreed with them in stating that it was in this sensorium that sympathy was effected, for they had suggested that the binding of certain nerves in common *fasciculae* was the cause.

These ideas of Vieussens and Willis were widely adopted, some authors (like Glaser) adding the cerebellum to the list, and others (like Schelhammer) criticizing Willis' speculation.

To the radiant emanations and concourse of particles of the parts of Willis' soul, and the mechanical flow of the Cartesian spirits was soon added the vibrations of Newton's aether. At the end of the *Principia* (1687)[54] Newton suggested that sensation and motion were owing to its vibrations in the solid nerves, to and from the brain. At the termination of the nerves was the *sensorium*, to which was in some way attached the soul, which, he told a friend, was incorporeal, living and intelligent. Whytt named Newton as an advocate of an extended soul, but Newton's remarks seem confined to the role of the aether. From the *Principia*, the questions subjoined

[51] D. Duncan, *Explication nouvelle et méchanique des Actions animals*, Paris, 1678.

[52] G. B. de Saint Romain, *La Science naturelle dégagée des Chicanes de l'école*, Paris, 1679. From L. Thorndike, *A History of Magic and Experimental Science*, 1923, vol. 8, p. 294.

[53] R. de Vieussens, *Neurographia Universalis*, Leyden, 1684, p. 125.

[54] K. D. Keele, op. cit., p. 88.

to the *Optica* (1704) and a conversation published in 1740,[55] it appears that the aether was a universal psychical as well as physical fluid, responsible for the nerve impulse and the presentation of sensation to the soul in the *sensorium*, by means of vibrations. The *sensorium* was certainly extended, and the mechanical vibrations of the aether within it would seem to argue an extended soul, but Newton does not appear to be specific upon this point. The aether is an agent of the soul, like animal spirits, but behaving like a *pneuma*.

Bontekoe[56] in 1698 had suggested a mechanism of sensation (from the nerves to the *sensorium* in the *corpus callosum*[57]) by means of vibrations or waves, probably under the influence of Huygens. Before being taken up by Hartley (see below), this idea was used also by Swedenborg in 1719.[58]

Towards the end of the century opinion inclined away from placing mental functions in structures within the brain, and many, agreeing with Steno[59] that Willis had been too speculative, favoured a more general placing of the soul in the substance of the brain. One of these writers was Humphrey Ridley who was inclined to be critical of authorities rather than promote the importance of his own ideas. He rejected the Cartesian system of the pineal as the seat of the soul, and also disagreed with Willis, Vieussens and Malpighi, whose structures serving functions of the soul within the brain were neither so clearly delimited as these had claimed, nor so justified by argument. The 'whole medullary part of the brain'[60] he said, was the common sensory in which the purely single soul performs the mental functions which are thus not distinct by seat.

As we have seen in the chapter on reflex action, observations by Redi, Baglivi, Caldesi, Preston and others showed that life could continue in the absence of the brain, and attention was drawn to the importance of the meninges, and of the spinal cord. Like Whytt, Ridley concluded from the evidence afforded by the survival of a decapitated tortoise, that the vital and involuntary motions were owing to the soul acting in a non-conscious way in the cerebellum and spinal medulla. These actions are 'irresistible' as Whytt's are obligatory.

The importance of the meninges, which impressed Baglivi, was associated with the idea that the brain was a gland, secreting the

[55] B. R., *Sir Isaac Newton's Account of the Aether*, 1740.
[56] K. D. Keele, op. cit., p. 88.
[57] G. Soemmering, *über das Organ der Seele*, Köningsberg, 1796, p. 33.
[58] G. Trobridge, *Swedenborg, Life and Teaching*, London, 1945, p. 64.
[59] N. Steno, *A Dissertation on the Anatomy of the Brain*, 1669, trans. G. Douglas, 1733, reprinted, Copenhagen, 1950, p. 11.
[60] H. Ridley, *The Anatomy of the Brain*, London, 1695, p. 190.

nervous spirits from the blood into the nerves. The meningeal membranes aided this flow by contraction. Antonio Nuck, who wrote a book on glands, the *Adenographia Curiosa et Uteri Foeminei Anatome Nova* of 1696,[61] held that the brain was such a gland, and dispensed its spirits from an organizing centre, the *promptuarium spirituum*, which was also the common sensory, and which he placed in the *centrum ovale*. Like other writers, he believed all the nerves terminated in this organ, to which the parallel fibres of the *corpus striatum* were conducting vessels. Typical of his time in these beliefs, Nuck also composed a suitable epitaph upon the system of Descartes, recalling Bartholin's lament for the liver. A fitting finale for the seventeenth century, it may be rendered thus:

VIATOR

Hold your ground.
With grave attention Behold
The buried Conarium
The body's chiefest Part, the
Seat of the Soul
the Pineal Gland.
Born and extinguished in this age,
Fame strengthened and
Opinion upheld its
Majesty and Splendour.
It lived until its
Aura as a divine Particle
Vanished, and the limpid Lymph
Fulfilled its place.

VIATOR
Depart without the gland.
Leave to others this Conarium
Lest posterity wonder at your
Ignorance.

Surveying his own century, Whytt could find little support for his ideas. The conceptions of the soul he attacked were already a little old-fashioned, so that the support he gained by these refutations was anyway granted him by the temper of the times; and the endorsement he sought elsewhere was sometimes a little strained.

[61] It was published in Leyden. The apostrophic epitaph is from p. 152.

Thus, after a final burst of unorthodoxy at the beginning of the century, no one would care to own that the soul was material, and Whytt was preaching to the converted. Perhaps, however, he felt that the coextensive soul was more open to suspicion of materiality than one unextended, and he is at pains to prove his point. Examine, he urges his readers, the letters written by Samuel Clarke to Henry Dodwell, wherein 'Perspicuity, Metaphysics and sound Philosophy are happily united'[62] and by which a dangerous and foolish heresy was blotted from the pages of the eighteenth century.

Dodwell, in fact, had done little more than to base his speculative theology upon Tertullian rather than St. Augustine, and was, perhaps, unprepared for the storm which blew up over his *Epistolary Discourse* of 1706,[63] by which he proved the soul to be naturally mortal, and raised up only by the pleasure of God. Prelates and philosophers rushed into print against him, Clarke[64] among them. Dodwell came back strongly with a *Preliminary Defence*,[65] aided by the support of Anthony Collins,[66] an advocate of 'natural' interpretations of religious questions. The publication of rival pamphlets continued until 1711,[67] and from this debate on mortality, we need only inspect (as Whytt suggested) Clarke's observations on the related state of materiality.

Clearly, a material soul is exposed to physical decay, an inevitable attribute of all matter, and so is suspect in regard to immortality. How, asks Clarke, can a system of matter ever achieve the capacity of thinking unless matter itself, in its smallest division was essentially conscious? No; the soul was immaterial and apart, acting through the material and unconscious brain.

When Whytt rejected the views of 'some modern materialists', who considered that the soul was a subtle substance circulating with the blood, he may have been thinking of William Coward, drawn by later observers into the Dodwell controversy. His *Second Thoughts Concerning the Human Soul* (1702) seems also to owe something to Tertullian. The soul is a 'divine afflatus'[68] breathed by God into Adam's lifeless frame, and propagated from generation to generation. Yet this was no *pneuma* or spirit, but a faculty by which matter could feel and live. Soul and life, said Coward, are

[62] R. Whytt, *An Essay on the Vital and Other Involuntary Motions of Animals*, p. 281.
[63] Published in London.
[64] S. Clarke, *A Letter to Mr. Dodwell*, London, 1706, and *A Defence of an Argument*, London, 1707.
[65] London, 1707.
[66] A. Collins, *A Reply to Clarke's Defence . . .*, London, 1707.
[67] Including Dodwell's *The Natural Mortality of the Humane Soul*, London, 1708.
[68] W. Coward, *Second Thoughts Concerning the Human Soul*, London, 1702, p. 107.

terms of equal meaning. Life was matter thus enlivened, and the soul was necessarily extended to all parts of the body, its nature in every part determined by the structure of that part. This superficial resemblance to Whytt's sentient principle is paralleled by Coward's declaration that the soul is a necessary agent, 'and not an intelligent act, power or principle'.[69] Thoughts were merely motions produced in the brain by the movements of the purely material spirits, and as such were liable to all kinds of change from a variety of physical causes: 'meats and drinks', exercise and damage.

In contradistinction to Clarke, and Whytt, the intellect was thus the product of active matter; it was the brain which thought. This may owe something to Locke, who had incautiously observed that God being omnipotent, it was within His power to give intellect to matter. It would have been as reasonable, observed a bitter defender of the faith, for Locke to have said it was in God's power to have made the moon out of green cheese 'and if he had said so it is very probable that Dr. Coward would have published a book to show that it was so made, and have call'd it his Second Thoughts of the Moon made of a Green Cheese.'[70]

Just as Whytt's sentient principle shows similarities to the coextensive soul of Epicurus and Lucretius, so the similar soul of Coward seems to show indebtedness to the ancient atomists. The blood, he observed, was the most proper subject for the afflatus to act upon, and it was by its circulation that life was most apparant. Being material, the soul perished with the body, and differed from that of Epicurus only in its ultimate share in the general resurrection. The comparison between the two authors was also made by the same outspoken critic of the materialists. Epicurus' doctrine was nothing inferior to Dr. Coward's, he said, an 'Oracle for Lack Wits'.[71]

Perhaps rather old-fashioned were the coextension and materiality pictured by J. Tabor. The soul was principally within the brain, but also it permeated the body, reaching every part like light, 'as if of its own substance',[72] and there it performed the offices of the senses and addressed itself to the functions of the body. Important among the latter were the processes of digestion in which Tabor's soul seems allied to the nutritive soul of the older philosophers. The analogy to light brings Willis to mind, but Tabor says his debt is to Hippocrates.

Among the last of the materialists is Swedenborg. His early

[69] Quoted by C. Fleming, *A Survey of the Search after Souls*, London, 1758, p. 61.
[70] B. Hampton, *The Existence of the Human Soul after Death*, London, 1711, p. 6.
[71] B. Hampton, op. cit., p. 27.
[72] J. Tabor, *Exercitationes Medicae*, London, 1724, p. 301.

ideas on the vibration theory of sensation were followed in 1739 or 1740 by his conception of the soul as material and circulating with the blood. The physiology of the *Economy of the Animal Kingdom* is firmly based in the seventeenth-century orthodoxy of animal spirits derived from the blood. In the blood was the 'most spirituous fluid', the 'essential vital principle . . . the soul'.[73] The spirit, separated from the blood in the brain, was propelled into the nerves by pulsation or 'animation' of the brain. This animation concerned the *animus*; the higher soul, immortal and rational, was the *mens*.

The corporeal soul was so essentially a part of matter that no body-soul problem arose and no difficulties of the Clarke-Dodwell-Coward kind were encountered. Like Coward's *afflatus*, this soul owed its characteristics to God, but to dispute whether the matter or its faculties were the soul would be needless sophistry, particularly as by Swedenborg's definition of matter (which did not include inertia) both materiality and immateriality were predicable of the soul.

In the section on the soul in the posthumously published parts of *The Animal Kingdom*, Swedenborg turned his attention to the rational soul. This was immaterial and was related most closely to the material *sensorium* in the brain. This soul was the 'form' of the body in the Platonic sense, and its operations, unusually, were located in the cortex as well as the medulla of the brain. In the cortex were the 'sensations of light, perception and understanding'.[74] All motions of fibres of the brain were movements of the 'medullary lake' of the soul.

After these authors, the material *anima* virtually became extinct, although Whytt considered it necessary to reject materiality in his considerations of the soul. All would have agreed with him: 'Some modern materialists have imagined the *anima* to be no other than a mere subtile kind of matter lodged chiefly in the brain and nerves and circulating with the grosser fluids: but such matter can no more be imagined the vital principle or source of animal life than the blood from which it is derived . . . mere matter is not endued with sense or perception . . . thought or reflection; not even fire, the most subtile.'[75]

With the disappearance of the materialists, three different schools of thought supplied the climate of opinion from which Whytt drew: the Stahlians, the mechanists and the followers of Willis. For all the soul was now single, immaterial and possessed of the properties

[73] G. Trobridge, op. cit., p. 68.
[74] E. Swedenborg, *The Soul, or Rational Psychology*, trans. F. Sewell, New York, 1900, p. 12.
[75] *Works*, p. 147.

of the lower souls. Generally, too, the immaterial soul, if extended, was as limited in that extension as the mechanists would limit it in action; coextension was as old-fashioned as the material soul to which it was best suited.

Since Asclepiades, many observers had attempted to demonstrate that the removal of a vital organ showed that the soul could not reside therein, and just as in the history of the reflex the removal or absence of the brain focused attention on the spinal cord, the same observation could be taken to point to the meninges as organs of importance. In examining a premature and monstrous infant which enjoyed a brief existence in the year 1709 in the absence of a brain, J. H. Vogli[76] and several Berlin physicians concluded that the meningeal membranes were of greater importance in sense and motion than the brain or spinal cord. Using this sort of evidence and that which had inspired Baglivi, Johann Daniel Gohl asserted, as Back had done, that the meninges were the *sensorium commune*. His *Insufficientia Cerebri* of 1732 argued that these membranes were the origin of the nerves (from Erasistratus) that they existed before the brain, that nervous spirits were the agents of sense and motion and that the medullary part of the nerves played no part in these processes. The brain was the 'instrument and minister' of the soul.

As for the soul itself, Gohl was a Stahlian. Its function was to regulate the body in health by control of secretion of humours and to guard against disease by characteristic reactions of the body to infection. All its actions, particularly the vital motions, were performed freely by the soul, which did not 'suffer itself to be kept in the bounds of necessary mechanism'. Tonus, that vital tension of the bodily fibres, was the *summum documentum* of the soul's action.

At the risk of upsetting the sequence of chronology, discussion of Stahl (he died in 1734) has been reserved, for it is through his 'school' that his name tangles with that of Whytt. Historically Stahl seems to fall into place after Paracelsus and Van Helmont,[77] but what debt he owes them is obscure.[78] He is best regarded as the leader of the animist reaction against the mechanism of Descartes, which has been mentioned above.

Stahl's soul was single, active and intelligent. Motion as a category, and more particularly direction, was almost a metaphysical concept to him: motion was inconceivable without direction and direction without purpose. The vivifying soul pursued this purpose and provided the means—motion—to achieve it.

[76] J. D. Gohl, *Insufficientia Cerebri ad Sensum et Motum Animalis Expenditur* Colberg, 1732, p. 49.
[77] A. Lemoine, *Le Vitalisme et l'Animisme de Stahl*, Paris, 1864, p. 7.
[78] L. J. Rather, 'G. E. Stahl's Psychological Physiology', p. 39.

This, opposing them, makes Whytt's, Haller's and the Cartesian scheme seem more allied. In all these the parts of the body were so arranged (Whytt's 'original constitution') and set up by God (whether animated or 'mechanical', parts were given the otherwise inexplicable power of motion by the Creator) that the same purpose was achieved without the necessary knowledge or concurrence of the soul.

This purpose was preservation of the body, and it has already been noted that in the confused area of physiology where knowledge of autonomic and reflexive actions grew out of 'vital', 'voluntary', 'involuntary' and 'sympathetic' actions, all, including Whytt, agreed that there were automatic actions instituted to protect the body. Stahl, on the other hand, claimed that even in these actions the soul acted as the result of reason, even though this might not be rendered to the consciousness.

The followers of Stahl constitute the first of the three schools of thought mentioned above. Commentators from Haller to Garrison have called Whytt a Stahlian, and yet Whytt poured his choicest scorn upon Stahl and his school. 'All motions proceed from the soul'; both Whytt and Stahl said this, and for this reason Haller grouped them together, with Gohl, Goelicke, and Nicholls. Certainly in an age of mechanism this phrase conferred an important distinction upon the physicians who uttered it, but it need not be emphasized how shallow a comparison between Stahl and Whytt must be.

Whytt was undoubtedly mortified when such comparisons were made. To have his ideas classed with 'the indeed extravagant notions of Stahl and his followers' kindled in him that asperity of which Haller complained. 'I have met with no author' observed Whytt of Frank Nicholls 'who has embraced the Stahlian doctrine with less reserve, or carried it to a greater height than a learned physician[79] in his late elegant Praelection *de anima medica*. . . . But, as this account of the agency of the soul, and of its power over the body, scarcely seems to demand an answer . . .'.[80]

Nevertheless, Whytt did answer it, and with a ready flow of elegant analogy that would have graced the arguments of Lucretius himself, who may indeed have inspired it:

. . . I shall only observe, that to imagine the soul should, with the wisest views and in the most skilful manner, at first form the body, (a work far above the efforts of human art and

[79] This is Pringle's tactful substitution for Nicholls' name, which appears in the original essay on the vital motions, but not in the collected *Works*.
[80] *Works*, p. 145.

contrivance!), and afterwards, when it is disordered, should, with the same skill and wisdom, often remedy the evil, and restore it to a sound state; but finding it in the end, or sometimes suspecting it only, to be no longer tenable or comfortable, should, instead of repairing, either whimsically or wisely desert it: to conceive, I say, of the soul as performing all this, without, in the meantime, being conscious of such intentions, or of the exertions of its power in pursuance of them, is at least as fanciful as to suppose, that an architect might raise a stately edifice, in which nothing should be wanting that could contribute either to its usefulness or ornament; that he might frequently repair such damages as it sustains from the weather, or from the decay of any of its materials; and at last apprehending it to be in danger of falling, might abandon it; without being conscious of ever having once exercised either his skill in contriving, erecting, and repairing it, or his prudence in quitting it, when, as he thought, it was ready to bury him in its ruins.[81]

The lecture *De Anima Medica* had been given to the Royal College of Physicians in 1748. Critics of the Stahlian school from Behrens to Cullen had pointed out that no medical judgement is possible of a freely-acting soul. Nicholls lays himself open to the same charge: 'How foolish and imprudent is the soul!'[82] he observes. Perverse and arrogant, it was a law unto itself, and followed no other rules. This contrast to Whytt's 'laws of union' is heightened by a later passage: although generally astute and skilful, pursuing the interests of the body in the wisest manner, its vagaries and whims are characteristic of a free soul which is not circumscribed 'by the sluggishness of matter, as a machine driven by weight, nor is it a necessary agent in a body irritated by a stimulus . . .'.[83] The 'necessary agent' and 'stimulus' must have seemed to Whytt like a personal rejection of his own ideas. Nicholls could possibly have seen Whytt's essay on the causes of circulation in the small vessels, where Whytt makes much use of the idea of a stimulus activating the contractility of the capillaries, but he could not have seen Whytt's treatise on the vital motions, published three years after Nicholls' lecture, in which the role of the sentient principle as a necessary agent was elaborated.

Of Stahl himself, Whytt observed: 'It is true that Stahl, by extending the influence of the soul, as a rational agent, over the

[81] *Works*, p. 146. This passage was 'genteel stricture' said the contemporary *Monthly Review*.
[82] F. Nicholls, Compare Lucretius, p. 105. *De Anima Medica*, London, 1773, p. 14.
[83] Ibid., p. 25.

body a great deal too far, has been the occasion why, for many years, it has been considered rather as a subject of ridicule, than deserving a serious answer.'[84]

The essential difference between the two doctrines was, of course, that Whytt believed the soul reasoned only in the brain, and elsewhere acted as a necessary agent: 'Nor can we consider the mind as acting either ignorantly or perversely, when it sometimes excites such motions in the body as increase its own pain, and, in the end, prove more hurtful than beneficial; for these motions do not proceed, as the followers of Stahl have imagined, from any rational views in the mind, or a consciousness that the welfare of the body demands them, but are an immediate consequence of the disagreeable perception which excites it into action.'[85]

The second school of thought facing Whytt was that composed of those who held a greater or lesser allegiance to Cartesian mechanism. At one extreme of this school was Yvo Gaukes,[86] who hoped to bring the precision of mathematics into medicine. His dissertation of 1712 translates the Cartesian mechanism into more anatomical terms, and answers some contemporary criticisms of mechanism.

The nervous spirits carried a 'radiation' of sense and motion across the ventricles to and from the pineal gland. In the same way as a ship moving through water, or a river flowing round an arch of a bridge leaves a 'radiation' or 'progressive motion', so did the pineal gland and nerves disturb the nervous spirit. In a round vessel, observed Gaukes, such radiations are reflected to and fro, until they meet each other; the impulse travelling along the nerves emitted such radiations upon its entry to the ventricles and these radiations of the flowing juice were reflected about from the surface of the ventricles until they came together in the round sinus, where, in the vascular plexus, hung the pineal gland. The resulting movement of this afforded sensation by a species of occasionalism; the movement was an 'intermediate motion' and the mind received corporeal appearances by a *voluntas divina*. In this way the pineal gland, being the last material link before the immaterial mind in the sequence of sensation, was the corporeal *sensorium*, while the mind, the last human member communicating to God, was the *sensorium spirituale*. Radiations flowing back again to the ventricles, having become modified by circumnavigating the pineal, occasioned

[84] *Works*, p. 140.
[85] Ibid., p. 520.
[86] Y. Gaukes, *Dissertatio ad Medicina ad Certitudinem Mathematicum Evahenda*, Amsterdam, 1712.

142

motion, by passing into the nerves. The pineal governed this motion as the wake of a stick held in running water can be accurately controlled by movements of the stick.[87]

The inclination of the age toward mechanism is seen in the doctrines of the Associationist philosophers. Locke's idea of Association was used by Hume to investigate mental phenomena with scientific principles, and Hartley took up in addition Newton's suggestions on the physiological role of the ether to produce an almost mechanical explanation of perception, which recalls that of Hobbes. To consider the details of this mechanism would be too great a digression, and we must be content to observe the consequences of it on Hartley's conception of the soul.

Hartley was aware of the difficulties of the relationship between an immaterial soul and vibrations of matter within the brain which were the means of perception, and to avoid the stigma of materialism, he made a pious but rather unscientific declaration: 'But to this I answer that I am reduced to the necessity of making a *postulam* at the entrance of my enquiries; which precludes all possibility of proving the Materiality of the soul from this theory afterward. Thus I suppose, or postulate, in my first proposition that sensations arise in the soul from motions excited in the medullary substance of the brain'.[88]

The vibrations were of the small 'and, as one may say, infinitesimal medullary particles'[89] and analogous to the motion of small bodies produced by heat. Although he could not derive a connection between vibration and sensation, Hartley thought it was sufficient to demonstrate that a connection existed. It was unimportant if the cause was physical (with the system of the schools) occasional (Malebranche) or an adjunct (Leibnitz). Whytt used the same argument, that it was enough to observe that an event inevitably followed another (his law of union) without finding a cause. The vibrations were maintained by the ether, and pursued their motions along solid rather than tubular nerves.

The seat of the soul varied according to the species of animal involved: 'The brain may therefore in a common way of speaking, be reckoned the seat of the sensitive soul or sensorium in Men and in those animals where the medullary substance of the nerves and spinal marrow is much less than that of the brain'.[90]

In lower animals the *sensorium* was wider spread, and using

[87] Ibid., p. 208.
[88] D. Hartley, *Observations on Man, his Frame, his Duty and Expectations*, London, 1749, vol. I, p. 511.
[89] Ibid., p. 11.
[90] Ibid., p. 31.

similar arguments to Whytt, Hartley even toyed with coextension: '. . . one may question, whether in animals of the Serpentine Form and those whose brains are comparatively small, and in all those of the polypose kind, the sensorium be not equally diffused over the whole medullary substance, or even over all the living parts'.[91]

These two passages recall Whytt's opinion: 'Nay, while, in man, the brain is the principal seat of the soul, where it most eminently displays its powers, it seems to exist or act so equally through the whole bodies of insects, and other animals of the lowest class, that its power or influence scarce appears more discernible in one part than another'.[92]

In general the medulla of the brain, spinal nerves and marrow, were the instruments of sensation and 'related' to the sensitive soul, just as the sense organs are to them, and thus 'we may conclude absolutely' that the *sensorium* of such animals (including man) is to be placed in the brain 'or even in the innermost regions of it'.[93] Haller, who described Hartley as placing it in the brain and spinal cord, seems only to have read the chapter headings.

Despite his disclaimer, Hartley engaged in speculation concerning the relationship between body and soul. He postulated an 'infinitesimal elementary body' between the soul and body, and that all changes occurring in the medulla of the brain had to be transmitted through this particle. Thus it could modify, by its character, any such vibration, and the changes in the soul arising from it. The increasing suspicion of the existence of nervous spirits encouraged the notion of an ethereal vibration. Battie, writing on insanity, explained it as a 'pressure' within the nerves which produced an alteration in the material particles of the nervous medulla and brain. Concerning this change, '. . . we have no idea whatever, either visible or intellectual, how and in what manner those particles are by such pressure, differently juxtaposited previously to the sensations thereby excited'.[94] Such pressure was the last in order of the known causes of sensation, the rest being 'mere conjecture'.

One of the effects of mechanism was to deprive the soul of its recently-acquired vegetative functions and relegate them to the machinery of the body. In this way the term 'soul' could be used synonymously with 'consciousness' by the middle of the eighteenth century, by which time too the Continental Rationalists were prepared to argue away the soul completely.

[91] Ibid., p. 31.
[92] *Works*, p. 202.
[93] D. Hartley, *Observations on Man*, p. 31.
[94] W. Battie, *A Treatise on Madness*, London, 1758, p. 25.

Thus La Mettrie (1748) extends mechanism to cover mental operations. Old arguments for the materiality of the soul are revived: what seem to be functions of the soul must be merely motions of matter as they are so readily affected by material causes; the souls (consciousness) of Englishmen, who eat too much under-done meat, are drawn to resemble those of the carnivorous animals whose diet they share.

La Mettrie is an eighteenth-century Asclepiades. Detached vital organs not only survive but also do not cause the immediate decease of the remainder of the body. Do the separated parts of an animal each contain a soul? No; the body is a machine, working in each of its parts, and the soul 'is but an empty word, of which no one has any idea, and which an enlightened man should use only to signify the part in us which thinks . . .'.[95] The list of examples and experi-ments he quotes is very similar to that used by Whytt, including Boyle's observations on insects, and heart tissue in an evacuated 'receiver'. In the observation on the decapitated fowl, Kaau, whom Whytt mentions, is replaced by 'a drunken soldier'. The other examples of excised parts surviving are similar, La Mettrie only adding that the dismembered parts of a polyp will regenerate. The whole body, then, is a machine, a machine 'which winds its own springs', and its excised parts have the same springs but cannot wind them, and so eventually die. These springs of life which maintain motion in an excised muscle constitute an 'innate force' possessed by every fibre, a mechanical force inherent in the very 'parenchyma' of the tissue. This force inheres in every tissue *accord-ing to its need*. In just the same way, the evidence of living dismembered bodily parts led Whytt to postulate a coextensive soul, differing in its locations, as a sentient and motive principle, and persuaded Haller that muscular tissue had a *vis insita*.

The brain is the 'mainspring' of the body and life, 'for the brain has muscles for thinking as the legs have muscles for walking'.[96] Here, at the termination of the nerves, is the *enormon*, which others would call the soul. More like Spinoza than Descartes, he avoids the body-soul problem by emphasizing the identity of thought and matter: matter is sentient, and reason is sentience perceiving itself.

The third and most important school of thought facing Whytt was derived ultimately from the doctrines of Willis. The soul Willis described survived as the orthodox opinion, with the important change that his lower, fiery soul disappeared, leaving its functions to the higher. Only briefly did it enjoy these privileges however,

[95] J. de la Mettrie, *Man a Machine, 1748*, trans., Illinois, 1961, p. 128.
[96] Ibid., p. 132.

145

for current physiology recalled them into the soul-free sphere of mechanism. As suggested above, the result of this was to equate 'soul' with consciousness rather in the modern manner, and by the middle of the century it was possible for Haller to argue against Whytt that simultaneous and co-ordinated motions could not proceed from the soul, as it was only capable of entertaining one idea at a time.

Before this, however, the extension of Willis's idea of a centralized soul had already created the climate of opinion that was to make Whytt's coextension look odd to his contemporaries. The cool but not discouraging light of reason of the eighteenth century was thrown upon the speculations of Willis by La Peyronie, whose dissertation of 1708 caused a stir of interest. He had systematically collected evidence from surgeons on the effects of wounds and diseases in the head. Large quantities of the cerebral cortex were often carried away or consumed by disease without loss of faculties; the pineal gland was sometimes putrified or totally wanting; the nates, testes, infundibulum, corpus striatum and cerebellum were all open to the same objections. There remains, he observed, the corpus callosum. Not only did La Peyronie employ systematic observations, but also experiment: in one case the removal of an abscess the size of an egg opened a cavity reaching to the corpus callosum, which, relieved of its burden, returned its owner to consciousness. By alternately filling and emptying the cavity of water from a syringe, it was found that the condition of the sufferer could be controlled at will. 'Voilà', he concludes, 'l'âme installée dans le corps calleux'.[97]

This corresponds to Willis' location of conscious perception, but is at odds with his placing of the *sensorium commune*, and with Vieussens, who had placed none of the faculties of the soul here. Continental authors inclined more to Vieussens than to Willis, and the problem of reconciling Vieussens to La Peyronie can be seen in Diderot or Camerarius;[98] even La Mettrie notes La Peyronie's work with approval.

La Mettrie links La Peyronie's name with Lancisi. Lancisi's dissertation on the seat of the soul (1712) employs older arguments on behalf of the corpus callosum. It was single, central, at the termination of the nerves and connected to most parts of the brain, particularly the septum lucidum, fornix and the 'secretory cortex'. Spirits from the latter were directed into the corpus callosum by the contractile meninges and this activity could be felt during periods

[97] Quoted from Diderot and D'Alembert, *Encyclopédie ou Dictionnaire raisonné des Sciences, des Arts et des Métiers*, Paris, 1751, vol. I, p. 341.
[98] E. Camerarius, *Eclecticae Medicinae Scripta*, Frankfurt, 1713, p. 21.

of protracted concentration. Thus the corpus callosum, embodying the whole personality of the soul was physically different in individuals, so much so that its varieties of shape were manifest to the exterior by the configuration of the bones of the cranium. The soul was present in some undeclared way at this 'certain common emporium of sensations'.[99]

A useful criticism and summary of doctrines of the location of the soul is found in Behrens' study on medical aspects of the rational soul (1720). Although this is the 'rational' soul, Behrens notes that his contemporaries add to it the faculties of the vegetative and sensitive souls—the process of assimilation we have met before. With La Peyronie and others, all the old seats of the soul are dismissed: pineal, meninges, nates and testes and cortex. Its location was dictated by anatomy. It had to be at the end of all the nerves, just as previous authors had said, yet these authors had been too speculative, too ready to assume that the corpus striatum, callosum, or centrum ovale were the sole termination of the nerves. No, said Behrens, all that could be said for certain was that the sensorium and attendant soul were *somewhere* within the medulla of the brain. This sensorial *meditullium* consisted of the corpus callosum, the corpora striata, the centrum ovale, and even the nates, testes and thalami nervorum opticorum.[100]

This caution was typical of the eighteenth century, and of the way Willis's ideas were forged into medical orthodoxy. Like other writers of his century, too, Behrens anticipates the passing of the soul from the realm of medicine. It is impossible, he observed, to be acquainted with the nature of the soul, but it is enough to know that it obeys certain laws in the body. The business of the physician is to establish these laws. What hope would there be for medicine if the soul behaved freely and unpredictably, as Stahl said? Whytt said much the same of the need and possibility of knowing the soul, and he rejected Stahl in similar terms.

Later speculative ideas in the fashion of Willis are not convincing. Astruc,[101] who held like Whytt that the nerves were unbranched from origin to termination and thus all sympathy was referable to arrangements within the sensorium, placed this sensorium in the corpus striatum where Cartesian reflections (angle of reflection

[99] J. M. Lancisi, *Dissertationes II. De Physiognomia. De Sede Cogitantis Animae*, Rome, 1713, p. 159.

[100] R. A. Behrens, *Considerationem Animae Rationalis Medicam ... examini submittit*, Leipzig, 1720, p. 20.

[101] J. Astruc, 'An Sympathia Partium a certa Nervorum Positura in Interno Sensorio?' (1736) in A. von Haller, *Disputationes Anatomicae*, Göttingen, 1746-51, vol. I, p. 473.

being equal to angle of incidence) of spirits took place. Others, like Musschenbroek (1740)[102] were more cautious: how could it be shown even that the nerves terminated, and were not recurrent canals? In such a case the concept of a sensorium at the joint termination of the nerves would be untenable. It is clear, he said that it is quite impossible to know where or how the soul joined the body.

[102] P. van Musschenbroek, *Oratio Inauguralis de Mente Humana semet Ignorante*, 1740, p. 14.

CHAPTER XI

The Soul in Physiology

In the previous chapters we looked at some of the historical antecedents of Whytt's idea of the soul in anatomical terms. By the middle of the eighteenth century the location of the soul was generally agreed upon, and the influence exerted upon Whytt by his contemporaries was in the realm of physiology. Some of the older notions of the part the soul played in these bodily processes have been looked at in relation to 'sympathy' and the reflex. Just as the key word of Whytt's anatomical statements concerning the soul was 'coextension', so his physiological concepts are summed up in his 'laws of union' of body and soul. This chapter concerns itself with the possible sources of these and their reception by contemporaries.

These laws which determined the behaviour of the soul may be formulated[1] as follows:

1. The soul must perceive what is presented to it.

2. Its function in each part of the body is strictly limited. In the nerves, for example, the soul is only capable of 'feeling'.

3. Further, the soul in different nerves is sensitive to different stimuli.

4. The motive soul in muscle reacts differently to a direct stimulus than to one arriving 'sympathetically' by way of a nerve.

5. These four laws and the predetermined behaviour of the soul in the spinal cord, the centre of sympathy, provide (*a*) a set of beneficial reactions to changing external circumstances, and (*b*) a mechanism of normal physiological processes. Both can occur unconsciously.

Whytt thus arrives at an animistic mechanism which is as rigidly determined as any system governed by purely mechanical laws. His scheme stands opposed to the Stahlian freely acting and conscious soul, and the surviving mechanism of the orthodox physician.

One of the sources of this idea is found in the notes[2] Whytt made from the lectures of Dr. Young, the 'empirick' who distrusted

---

[1] Whytt himself did not draw up such a list of laws. They are derived principally from his essay on the vital motions, and to a lesser extent from his observations on sensibility and irritability.

[2] R. Whytt, *Notes on Dr. Young's Lectures* (dated 1766), in the Library of the Royal College of Physicians, Edinburgh, (not catalogued).

elaborate schemes of physiology. Mechanism is an incomplete explanation of sensation or motion; it is indeed only a description of observables, and in the generation of sensation in the brain from a disturbance in the nerves little could ever be observed. 'Mechanical connections are finite', wrote Whytt, 'and must at last terminate in a first cause'.[3] Animism was the simplest explanation of the process of sensation, where 'it would be ridiculous to ask after further mechanism'. Yet the disturbance in the sensory nerves was necessarily perceived by the soul in the brain—the first of the laws of union—for 'perhaps this is as particular and constant a law as the loadstone always attracts iron'.[4] As with sensation, so with muscular motion. What are the observables of contraction? Neither Keill, Mayow, Bernouille, Steno, Willis nor Boerhaave ever observed the spirits, acids and alkalis, ethers or fermentations which they had postulated. These 'mechanical' changes, Whytt clearly infers, *should* be visible; more agreeable to the lack of observables is an 'incorporeal Faculty' residing in the muscle. This is as near as Whytt comes in these early notes to his later concept of the soul. The term 'animism' is used above only as the most convenient expression of Whytt's antagonism to mechanism; his 'first cause' at this early date could equally well be God.

One of the authors from whom Whytt quotes is Alexander Stuart.[5] Whytt, if indeed he went to St. Andrews, may have there come under the influence of Stuart, who in turn had also been to Leyden. There he published an inaugural dissertation on the structure and motion of the muscles (1711). Stuart was a determined anti-mechanist. Like Willis, Ridley and Vieussens, his authorities, he recognized the participation of the soul even in the various kinds of involuntary motions. In these, unlike its action in voluntary motions, the soul did not act freely but was bound by laws. One of these laws of union was that the conscious part of the soul could not directly influence the motions of the vital parts, and another was that some vital activities must *always* be affected indirectly by voluntary motion, as the beating of the heart increases with exercise.

Whytt, however, was only expressly concerned with Stuart's anatomical ideas. Stuart was particularly interested in the nerves: he thought they contained a watery fluid,[6] like Whytt held that they were unbranched from origin to termination, and believed that the

[3] Ibid., p. 431.
[4] Ibid., p. 467.
[5] A. Stuart, *Dissertatio Medica Inauguralis de Structura et Motu Musculari*, Leyden, 1711.
[6] A. Stuart, 'Experiments to prove the existence of a fluid in the nerves', *Phil. Trans.*, 1731-1732, *37*, 324.

variety of bodily motions proceeded from the activity of their distal ends, which thus played their part in constituting the *sensorium:* this, Whytt said, was a kind of coextension. It is unlikely that Whytt would not also have noticed the physiological implications of this coextension, which carry the germ of his own idea of laws of union of body and soul. By means of this diffuse *sensorium*, continued Stuart, the *Imperium* of the soul was carried over the body, and here the soul either acted freely or was bound to act and feel through necessity.

At the centre of Leyden was Whytt's teacher, the great Boerhaave who spoke of 'laws of union' when motions are 'reflected' at the *sensorium* without the knowledge of the soul (but not in its absence). Surrendering some of the soul's lower activities to mechanism, Boerhaave differed profoundly from Whytt in virtually equating 'soul' with consciousness; nevertheless body and soul were bound by at least the law that certain states of the body are inevitably associated with certain ideas in the mind.[7] The mind must, in a word, perceive what is presented to it: Whytt's 'first' law.

A previous teacher of Whytt had been the elder Monro, who held that an obligation existed between soul and body in states of emergency; for example, the soul was bound to determine the removal of a limb from a source of pain, if severe.[8]

What Boerhaave had said was repeated by his successor Gaub,[9] whose textbook Whytt adopted for teaching purposes toward the end of his life. For Gaub even the vital motions came, however distantly, under the influence of the soul, but this was no freely acting arbitrary Stahlian soul, for Gaub attacked the Stahlian 'house of the soul' in a way which recalls Whytt's rejection of Nicholls. It may indeed have inspired it, or perhaps they both had read the same classical author.

Gaub held that the body contained two agents of arousal, a corporeal and a mental *enormôn*. These were responsible for movement of the body. The corporeal *enormôn*, the intermediary between mind and body, was located in the nerves and so was present like Whytt's sentient principle, in excised muscles, which it similarly enlivened. In the normal physiological processes of involuntary action, this agent of arousal was governed by laws not ultimately derived from the mind.

[7] H. Boerhaave, *De Morbis Nervorum*, Frankfurt and Leipzig, 1762, p. 436. The same idea is expressed in his *Institutions* (from W. Cullen, *Works*, Edinburgh, 1827, p. 20).

[8] F. Fearing, op. cit., p. 104.

[9] L. J. Rather, *Mind and Body in Eighteenth-Century Medicine*, London, 1965, has a good account of Gaub's views.

151

Gaub's rejection of the Stahlian soul (in an essay of 1747) is paralleled by Behrens, who said that the concept of the freely-acting soul was dangerous to medicine. Again, the conclusion is the not infrequent idea that the soul is bound to the body by laws. As Whytt shows so well, this is a fertile reconciliation of the animist and mechanist schools. Like other writers, Behrens announced only one law, that the soul must perceive what was presented to it, and that its affections were necessarily translated into motions of the body. Haller[10] points to the fact that the soul is obliged to perceive the 'corporeal species' which, belonging to the body, are also the only means the soul has of performing the mental faculties; by these the soul is strictly bound to the body. As this leads Haller to deny that the complex vital motions arise from the soul (which could entertain only one idea at a time), we may assume it had little influence upon Whytt. Haller repeated the argument in the controversy with Whytt.

These few suggestions concerning the origins of Whytt's 'laws of union' are sparse enough; the missing ingredient lies in the unique property of Whytt's sentient principle, which the souls described by these authors did not have: coextension. The writers who had favoured a coextensive soul were (in spirit at least) pre-mechanist and un-influenced by the idea of laws of union (with the possible exception of the limitation of function by want of organs imposed upon the soul of the ancient atomists as it pervaded the body). Whytt was in a position to combine both ideas, coextension and laws of union, in a fruitful amalgam.

We are thus brought back to coextension as the key to Whytt's concept of the soul, and we may usefully examine the reasons which first led him to this opinion, and from this opinion to his other laws of union.

The primary of these was the fact that an excised portion of an animal survived its separation from the greater whole. This observation had caused trouble from Aristotle and Asclepiades to Harvey and Haller, and in the eighteenth century had given rise to such different conclusions as those of La Mettrie, Haller and Whytt. Whytt's strong belief that no arrangement of matter could ever generate motion, which had caused him to fill out his notes on Young's lectures with speculations of his own, convinced him now that it was indeed the soul which caused the isolated muscle to twitch, just as it had made it contract in the body. The soul must therefore be extended to all living parts.

---

[10] A. von Haller, *First Lines of Physiology*, (reprint of the 1768 translation of the 1747 ed.), New York, 1966, vol. 2, p. 46.

This conclusion brought difficulties. How could an immaterial soul have extension as an attribute? Was it as divisible as the body through which it was extended? These old problems were particularly relevant to Whytt's unique immaterial coextension, and it must be admitted that he arrived at no very satisfactory answer. With Gassendi, he argued that the soul, universally acknowledged to be at the termination of the nerves, *must* be extended, as the nerves were of irreducible diameters and the soul acted simultaneously, therefore, at different places. A simple extension of this argument accounted for coextension, but still did not explain how extension, a property of matter, could be an attribute of an immaterial soul. Still less happy is his attempt to avoid making the soul divisible on the division of the body by emphasizing its immateriality. His arguments will be inspected more closely in relation to the criticisms of his contemporaries, it sufficing here to say that in Whytt's view these problems were unduly metaphysical for a physician, it being enough that the results of the soul's activity were predictable, for the more profound relationships of body and soul were unfathomable.

His arguments, therefore, that the soul is coextensive were based on observation and experiment of a physiological nature rather than scholastic logical ingenuity. He listed the observations he thought were most persuasive of coextension:

1. A frog was decapitated by Kaau and lived for half an hour. This was an experiment repeated many times by Whytt. Both halves of a bisected frog lived for the same time.
2. Kaau cut the head off a young cock, 'as he was running with great eagerness for his food; (he) went on in a straight line for twenty three Rhineland feet, and would have continued had he not met an obstacle which stopt him'. Bacon, noted Whytt, had a similar story about an ostrich decapitated by an arrow of a Roman emperor.
3. A viper without its head and entrails moved towards its habitual hiding place.
4. Boyle showed that a viper without its skin, head or heart will move for at least a day and is sensible of punctures. He also showed that female butterflies copulate and lay eggs after the loss of their heads.
5. Redi extracted the brain of a tortoise through a hole in the skull: 'immediately after the loss of its brain, it shut its eyes, nor ever opened them ever more, but continued to move and walk about until the time of its death'. It survived the operation six months.

6. A decapitated tortoise, allowed to bleed, lived for twenty-three days, during which time the heart continued to beat, and the feet retained sensitivity.

Whytt mentioned elsewhere that pigeons of Baglivi lived for several hours while destitute of brain. However, Baglivi seems to be referring to an experiment performed by someone else: '. . . adding anatomical experiment that is known to everyone, that birds (such as pigeons) although their brains have been removed will not only live for several hours, but also fly'.[11]

Whytt concluded (as Aristotle had done) that animals with diffuse nervous systems survive mutilation more readily, the faculties of the soul being less pronounced or localized. In these as in others, *all* motions proceeded from the soul:

> If the motions of a tortoise after decollation (35), or the loss of its brain (34), cannot proceed from mere mechanism, but must be undoubtedly ascribed to the living principle which was the cause of its motions in a sound state; and, if the same is true of the actions performed by butterflies after the loss of their heads (33); it must follow, that the motions and other signs of life which are observed in the body and limbs of a frog for above half an hour after its head is cut off (29), are to be attributed to the sentient principle, to which its motions and actions were owing when in an entire state; and if so, then the motions of this body when divided into two parts must also be referred to the same cause, since they are of a like kind, although of shorter duration.[12]

If two halves of an animal are animated by the soul, then so must be an excised muscle. To deny this 'would be to neglect the strongest analogy'. It could not be objected that the animal should feel pain when its excised member is irritated, if that member is animated by the same soul, for Whytt had pointed out that nerves are the sole organs of sensation (and retain this power out of the body) and these are cut off from the brain, the sole organ of consciousness. There would be, in the nerves of the excised, irritated part a 'simple sensation' as in oysters and other animals without brains and these nerves excite the muscles to contract. This is localized 'pain', which if not conscious, does exist in peripheral situations, and which recalls ideas of the ancient atomists and their later followers, such as Gassendi.

[11] Baglivi, *Opera Omnia*, Leyden, 1704, preface, p. 11.
[12] *Works*, p. 205. The numbers within brackets are Whytt's references to his own paragraphs.

Whytt decided that the best method of determining whether something was alive, that is, 'animated' or possessed of a soul, was to observe if it attempted to avoid that which pained or damaged it. Decapitated vipers clearly did this for at least three days: they were alive, 'and endued with feeling, i.e. animated by a sentient principle. And as the muscular parts of these creatures move after being cut in pieces, and are sensible of punctures, it also follows, that they continue still to be animated.'[13]

The soul, then, was coextensive. It was also single, for the *anima* of animals was no more than an undeveloped *animus* of man. Many actions previously thought proper to the *anima* could be taken over by the *animus* and vice-versa; the separate *anima*, with its connotations of materiality, was unthinkable; the one, as Lucretius had said, was in fact a faculty of the other.

Coextensive, single, the soul was necessarily limited in function to the tissue it occupied:

As the soul seems to imagine, judge, reason and remember in the brain only; why may it not have in the various other parts of the body, such feelings or powers as are necessary for carrying on their several functions? In particular why may it not have, in the muscular fibres, the power of simple sensation and of beginning motion? . . . the soul is equally present in the extremities of the nerves through the whole body as in the brain. In those it is only capable of feeling or simple sensation; but in this it exercises the powers of reflex consciousness and reason. When the communication of any part with the brain is cut off, the simple sensation or feeling in such a part is no longer perceived by the soul in the brain; and therefore is not attended by reflex consciousness . . .[14]

Coextension, singleness, local and limited function: from these observations, Whytt elaborated his 'laws of union' of body and soul. An excised muscle invariably contracted upon a stimulus as necessarily as a disturbance in a sense organ was perceived by the soul in the brain. This is what we have called the first of the laws of union:

The mind therefore, in carrying on the vital and other involuntary motions, does not act as a rational but as a sentient principle; which without reasoning is as certainly determined by

13 Ibid., p. 206.
14 Ibid., p. 287.

an ungrateful sensation or stimulus affecting the organs to exert its power in bringing about these motions, as is a scale which by mechanical laws turns with the greatest weight.[15]

The 'second law' follows directly from coextension: the function of every organ and tissue is an expression of the activity of the soul, which is thus limited in that tissue or organ. Matter enables the soul to work:

> It cannot well be objected here, that we describe the intelligent powers of mind to the bodily organs, for as the best musician cannot make the flute give the sound of the violin, or a harpsichord that of a French horn, nor without these several instruments produce their sounds and notes at all; in a like manner the soul, in its present state can only exercise its rational powers in the brain; it can only taste in the tongue, smell in the nose, see in the eyes, hear in the ears and feel hunger in the stomach. But although the imagination, memory and rational power depends upon the brain, smelling on the nose, seeing on the eyes and hearing on the ears, yet these organs neither taste, see or hear, but only that living sentient principle which animates them.[16]

This is directly opposed to the opinion of Coward and other materialists who had said that the soul enables *matter* to be sensitive and motive.

Such is the nature of the sentient faculty in the nerves (by the 'original constitution') that it is sensitive to a limited range of stimuli. Light only can awake the sensitive function of the optic nerves, and sound those of the ear; air produces a feeling of ease in the lungs but of pain in the stomach, while the opposite is true of food. This, anticipating the doctrine of the Specific Energies of Nerves,[17] is the third law. Each nerve may vary quantitatively but not qualitatively in its sensitivity; those of the heart may be rendered more sensitive by disease or mental states, resulting in a higher pulse rate. This law is so rigid that the increased heartbeat may endanger the safety of the body itself.

The excised muscle which exemplifies the first of these laws alternatively contracts and relaxes at a direct stimulus. In its original situation in the body, a natural direct stimulus has the same effect, while a stimulus relayed through the sympathetic centre

15 Ibid., p. 152.
16 *Works*, p. 288.
17 See above, p. 39-40, 82.

of the spinal cord by the nerves may produce a steady contraction by its different action upon the sentient principle: the 'fourth law'.

In the spinal marrow and that part of the brain unconcerned with initiating voluntary actions, the sentient principle is so arranged in the original constitution of soul and body that incoming sensory impressions are translated into motor activity best designed to preserve the body: the decapitated frog withdraws its damaged foot. Through this centre of sympathy also, as in the 'fourth law', the same process, designed to rid the body of an unpleasant stimulus, are performed normal bodily processes: a muscle stimulated upon its surface is thrown into alternate contractions which are best suited to remove the offending cause and in the same way the heart is repeatedly stimulated by the continued presence of the blood. Likewise the small vessels in inflammations, the guts, lungs and gonads are all stimulated by their contents. When, on the other hand, the stimulus originates more distantly and is relayed through a sympathetic centre, the physiological process is often best served by a steady contraction, as of the diaphragm in defecation from a stimulus arising in the rectum. The direction in which such a nervous impression is returned or 'reflected' from the sympathetic centre is always as constant, motor to sensory, as its force: in simple cases the extent of reaction is proportional to the extent of stimulus. This constancy, with these other considerations, we may group together as the 'fifth law'.

These laws were instituted in the body by God, and not imposed upon the soul by itself, as the Stahlians imagined. Likewise the soul itself was a gift of the Author of Nature, but apparently not a direct gift: animals occupied a mid-point in creation between wholly corporeal substances and beings which were immaterial intelligences. It was from the latter that animals derived their 'sentient and rational' powers, and the souls of animals, Whytt several times remarks, differ only in degree from those of men. This element of Platonism in Whytt's thought has already been noted (p. 99).

Correspondingly, upon death, the soul does not return at once to its Maker. Decapitation of animals or man (the argument is the same) is not instant death, but is irremediable. A laboratory animal can be drawn and quartered, yet death of its parts is not the immediate consequence of the 'death' of the whole; for many hours, even days, motions can be produced by stimulation of isolated muscles. Stimulation can equally recover the lives of animals or even men, who, trapped and frozen by snow, have ceased to breathe or exhibit a pulse. It is more likely that such stimuli reawaken the soul than recall it: was it possible that they 'could, as it were, by some magic charm, have called it back from distant regions?'[18]

No; stoppage of the heart is not death, but the first stage in the quiescence of the soul.

Whytt's doctrines were not enthusiastically received by his contemporaries. Total animism had gone out of fashion with Stahl, and coextension was even older. The verdict, indeed, of historians (of those, at least, who make any mention of him) has generally been that Whytt was a disciple of Stahl. This opinion probably derives ultimately from Haller, who, as we have seen, describes Whytt as a Stahlian 'inasmuch as he derives all motions from the soul'. Thus, in his review of Whytt's essay on animal motions (1752) Haller observes that nothing could be more specious than to attribute all motions to the activity of the soul. In addition he complains of Whytt's lack of candour, his destructive criticism, and Stahlian asperity. In his first publication (in the same year) on the sensitive and irritable parts of the body, Haller accused Whytt of subscribing to an opinion favouring divisibility of the soul, and was equally critical in the 1756 French treatise on the subject. The *Apologia* against Whytt groups him with Stahl, as does the *Elementa Physiologiae*. The opinion is repeated in the *Bibliotheca Anatomica* (see chap. 6). It is perhaps hardly surprising in the face of all these works of Haller that the notion of Whytt as a Stahlian should have survived.

Haller disagreed with Whytt not only in believing that some animal motions were independent of the soul, but also in his location of that soul. His views are probably most characteristic of the eighteenth century in general, and with this double parentage, they were the most damaging criticisms of Whytt's scheme.

Haller recognized, as La Peyronie had done, that the most convincing arguments were based on experiment and observation. His problem was simplified because he was dealing with the single rational soul that had consciousness as its chief if not its only characteristic: he argued firmly that the soul could not be in the spinal medulla, as damage inflicted on it did not affect integrity of mind. It need not be emphasized how differently Whytt interpreted damage to the spinal medulla, his sympathetic centre.

Similarly, said Haller, the cerebral cortex could not be the seat of the soul, as it was often wounded without loss of mental faculties. There remained the cerebral medulla, to which also pointed other evidence: it was the termination of the nerves, and convulsions followed from its irritation. Here was the extended *sensorium commune*, to which was joined in an unknowable fashion the un-

[18] *Works*, p. 201.

158

extended immaterial soul. In the *First Lines of Physiology*, Haller thought that the *sensorium* could be further limited to the corpora striata, thalamus, pons, and the medulla oblongata and cerebelli. By the time he wrote the 'conjecturae' in the fourth volume of the *Elementa Physiologiae*, he had changed his mind, and rejected all schemes limiting the *sensorium* to anything less than the whole of the cerebral medulla. He almost regretfully abandoned the idea that the cerebral localization of senses involved the roots of the corresponding sensory nerves. In these conjectures[19] Haller gives a useful summary of ideas on the seat of the soul, dismissing Whytt in the usual way.[20]

If Whytt was a Stahlian for Haller's purposes, the Stahlians, whom Whytt rejected with an asperity as great as that he turned on Haller, understood the situation rather better, and equally rejected Whytt. Typical of these was Porterfield, Whytt's colleague. 'Laws of union' were nonsense, said Porterfield; the soul was free to act as it chose, and was responsible in that capacity for all the actions of the body. Even the vital motions were originally voluntary, and only by 'use or custom' became fixed in pattern.[21]

For this reason, and because the soul was *not* extended to all parts of the body (said Porterfield) the soul was not limited in any way: 'And with respect to the soul's exercising different faculties in different parts of the body, this also seems to me to be extremely unphilosophical, for the whole soul is but one, and this one whole soul has not the same powers here and other powers there, but all its powers are powers of the whole and all its actions are actions of the whole; and this one whole soul exercises all its powers and faculties in that the whole place in which it is.'[22]

This opinion recalls the *tota in toto* argument of the middle ages. No such thing as localized pain could exist: the all-conscious soul, to which Whytt's 'simple sensation' or unconscious perception of a distant part of the body was quite foreign, was seated in the brain and did not extend peripherally to account for such sensation; how otherwise could Porterfield feel an itching sensation in the space once occupied by his ankle, now amputated? The coextensive soul, he forthrightly declared, implied divisibility, a supposition 'much more unaccountable than the phenomena themselves'. 'The natural and plain consequence of this indivisibility of the soul is,

---

[19] A. von Haller, *Elementa Physiologiae*, vol. 4, p. 392.

[20] Ibid., p. 394.

[21] 'In all this (the blink reflex) there is nothing of intrinsic necessity; the mind is at absolute liberty to act as it pleases'. The soul 'imposed a law upon itself' to obtain the most beneficial results. (From Fearing, *Reflex Action*, p. 104).

[22] W. Porterfield, *A Treatise on the Eye*, Edinburgh, 1759, vol. 1, p. 369.

that it cannot continue present with all the parts of the body after they are separated, and consequently this hypothesis ought to be laid aside as repugnant to that Oneness and indiscernibility of the soul, of which we have so many irrefragable proofs.'[23]

Whytt had anticipated such a criticism, and argued that the soul was not divisible, for a substance so 'perfectly and essentially one' could not be divided by physical separation of the parts to which it relates. As the Deity is present all the time in the infinitely distant parts of the universe, without being divisible, 'so, may not the souls of animals be present everywhere in their bodies, actuating and enlivening, at the same time, all their different members? Nay, further, when the fibres and threads connecting some of these parts are divided, may not the soul still act in the separated parts, and yet be only one mind?'[24]

In reconciling the extension, immateriality and indivisibility of God, Whytt owns his debt to the Scholastics, whose argument, and its application to the similar problem of the soul, we have already looked at. Whytt also (in the quotation above) transfers the logic from God to the soul, but thought that the Scholastics had said that as the soul was not extended in space, it occupied an indivisible point. He rejects this as he does the Cartesian scheme.

In other quarters Whytt's ideas were better received. James Johnstone's interest in sympathy led him to attribute much the same characteristics to the ganglia as Whytt gave to the spinal cord: they constituted a sympathetic centre, automatic but not mechanical, outside the rational powers of the soul.[25] In making experiments on decollated frogs, Johnstone[26] owned his debt to Whytt and expressed sympathy with his doctrines. Cullen, Whytt's colleague and successor, also speaks well of the latter's ideas, but otherwise Whytt seems to have fallen rapidly into obscurity.

[23] Ibid., vol. 1, p. 368.
[24] *Works*, p. 203.
[25] J. Johnstone, 'History of a foetus born with an imperfect brain', *Phil. Trans.*, 1767, *57*, 118.
[26] J. Johnstone, 'Experiments in support of uses ascribed to the nerves', *Phil. Trans.*, 1770, *60*, 30.

CHAPTER XII

The Demise of the Soul

The advance of physiology after Whytt was an erosion of the concept of soul. Before Descartes, the three souls of Aristotelian physiology were the causes of all motions of the body. All involuntary and vital motions were the functions of the lower souls, and as consciousness was an attribute only of the highest soul, there was no difficulty in explaining what part consciousness played in such motions: it was generally agreed to be very small.

The difficulty increased as the lower souls were assimilated into the upper (consciousness seeming a chief property of the amalgam) and when Descartes abolished the lower souls and relegated their functions to mechanism it became acute; not, of course in the Cartesian scheme itself, which was consistent but not widely adopted, but in the great influence it had among those who were in no great haste to dismiss the soul from physiology.

Thus the reflex action described by Willis was just as inevitable as that of Descartes, but not mechanical, as the soul took part in it. Here, then, the soul is treated in a new way. That the vital and involuntary motions should be as automatic as seemed desirable after Descartes, the soul was obliged to act in a certain way. (Here we may see the origin of Whytt's laws of union.) The difficulty became pronounced as it was realized that the soul that was thus constrained was the conscious and rational soul, which did not seem at all to be obeying laws; nor did it, indeed, seem to play *any* part in the vital motions. Whytt and others made use of the concept of 'unconscious sensation' to explain the soul's participation, while others like Haller invented mechanical forces or arrangements of parts to explain the vegetative and animal faculties as Descartes had done, leaving the soul a pure *animus*.

This erosion of the lower powers of the soul had been helped on its way by Boerhaave, who had formulated mechanical theories of the action of the heart and of respiration, and aided by Haller who tackled the basic question of muscular motion. The *vis insita* he attributed to the muscular 'glue' owed none of its capacity to move to the soul, a word he used in the same way as 'mind'. 'The heart and intestines, also some organs of the venereal appetite are governed by the *vis insita* and stimuli. These powers do not arise from the

161

will. . . . It is so certain that motion is produced by the body alone, that we cannot even suspect any motion to arise from a spiritual cause, except that which the will seems to excite in animals'.[1]

Another physiological concept which robbed the soul of some of its powers was the developing idea of 'sympathy'. To some extent, with its occult and independent causes, sympathy had always been free of the soul, and few of the many mechanisms proposed in the eighteenth century to explain its widely-accepted powers of bodily co-ordination owed anything to the soul. As the reflex removed the soul from many external actions so sympathy rendered it unnecessary in the management of the vital motions of the viscera.

Perhaps James Johnstone best demonstrates this tendency. The ganglia, he said (which were now coming to be recognized as typical of nerves concerned in sympathy) existed for the very purpose of preventing the action of the soul reaching the viscera, which were thus protected against whims of the will.[2] Others, like Supprian[3] and perhaps most orthodox physicians, recalled Willis's doctrine that the vagus and 'intercostal' nerves to the viscera arose from a part of the brain (here the medulla of the cerebellum) where the soul did not exert judgement. Likewise the sympathy experienced by many organs served by branches of these nerves was effected by the common membrane surrounding such branches at their origin, and owed nothing to the soul.

The very difficulty of discovering how body and soul were related encouraged the erosion of the powers of the latter, and here Whytt's laws of union helped to retain the concept of the soul. It is a remarkable fact that English (and here we must make it 'British') science in the eighteenth century moved forward in happy conjunction with religious faith while elsewhere it often encouraged scepticism or atheism.[4] This is reflected in attitudes toward the soul. Only European philosophers and physicians could whittle away its forces so readily, or contemplate its complete abolition.

For Descartes it had been a mere adjunct and for La Mettrie 'an empty word'. Haller banned it from all motion except that generated by the will, and Tissot[5] observed that the body could live without it. There were Germans who Behrens was too ashamed to

---

[1] A. von Haller, *First Lines of Physiology*, p. 196.

[2] J. Johnstone, 'Essay on the use of the ganglia of the nerves', *Phil. Trans.*, 1764, *54*, 177.

[3] F. L. Supprian, *Dissertationem Inauguralem Medicam, quae Medicinam absolute debere esse Philosophum praecipue ex Mirifica Cerebri structura*, Magdeburg, 1745, p. 37.

[4] B. Willey, *The Eighteenth Century Background*, Peregrine Books, 1962, pp. 47, 49.

[5] In the preface to Haller's *A Dissertation on the Sensibility and Irritability of the Parts of Animals*, 1755. (See p. 63).

name, because they had declared the soul did not exist. 'A little philosophy may dispose some men to Atheism,' said Whytt, echoing the opinion of his countrymen, 'but a more extensive knowledge of nature, will surely have the contrary effect.'[6]

Nevertheless, the central position of the soul as he conceived it in physiology obliged Whytt to circumscribe its activities by laws as strict as those governing mechanical systems. This is another kind of limitation or erosion which in fact reduced the concept of soul to that of *vital force* (except of course in the brain).

The result of this was the same as the result of Haller's thinking, or of that of other mechanists. For Whytt progress in physiology would have meant the discovery of new laws of union, while for Haller the same laws would be attributable to a mechanical arrangement of parts. Whytt had said that there was no need to enquire after the nature of the soul, it being necessary only to be certain of the manifestation of its activity in matter. *This* behaviour of matter was indistinguishable in practice from that of Haller, but it always retained a notion of the soul, which many of Whytt's countrymen preferred.

After these different kinds of erosion, the idea of soul acquired the meaning we have for it now: it is almost a synonym for 'mind', in a word, the old *animus*. It has been mentioned that Haller and others were using the word in this sense in the eighteenth century, and this gave rise to much of the confusion and misunderstanding which attended the debates on the soul between Whytt, Haller and the Stahlians. As Haller quite rightly suggested, the whole argument centred round the definition of 'sensation'. Haller would not accept unconscious sensation of the sort that Whytt used to explain the local sensitivity of parts of the body. When Whytt elaborated this to a quasi-mechanical sympathy to explain co-ordinated and simultaneous motions, Haller objected that simultaneous motions could not be owing to the soul, as the soul was capable only of perceiving one thought at a time. This suggests that Haller could not, rather than would not, understand unconscious sensation.

The Stahlians occupied a different territory. The soul, they said, was always conscious and acting for the best, but *did not* always share this consciousness with the owner of the soul. 'Sensation', then, could have three very distinct meanings, a confusion not helped by the different Latin styles adopted by different authors.

If, observed Haller, attempting to sort out the elements of the problem, *sensatio* is simply a physical disturbance in the nerves, then sensation would be excited everywhere, 'but if it is true that

[6] *Works*, p. 208.

163

to feel is the prerogative of the soul, and signifies a change within it',[7] then *sensatio* must be confined to the brain, the nervous disturbance being a mere physical *pressio*. Thus he admits of nothing between sensation and physical motion. Other authors employ *sensus* to indicate a non-physical disturbance in the nerves which there does not blossom out into *sensatio*, much as Whytt's unconscious sensation remains limited.

Whytt was the last of the animists. Lines of physiological research and the science itself progressed on smaller fronts, by asking answerable questions: it was no longer possible to conceive of a system of physiology *de novo*. Yet this progress could emerge from Whytt's founding stones as much as from Haller's, and we have already observed that their ideas were *in practice* similar. (Whereas their differences over the extent of sensibility in the body were very real in practical terms.) Thus the nature of the *vis insita* was just as obscure to Haller as the soul and its energy in the muscle were to Whytt. In neither case did this ignorance preclude the possibility of further illumination by observation and research: it was useless, said Whytt, only to enquire into the *nature* of the soul, and not its laws of union. The adoption of such a policy would keep the soul out of the way in further physiological enquiries.

Yet Haller's mechanical *vis insita* did not fill the gap left by thus keeping the soul out of sight, and the same complexity of living things which had made Whytt elaborate his notion of the soul produced a number of theories of vitalism in the nineteenth century. The opposition to mechanism remained, and indeed, still does.

It is difficult to trace Whytt's influence. Vestiges of his doctrine may be found in his own university for a few years after his death but in general his old opponent Haller had the last word. Not only was Haller's physiology more immediately acceptable and available to a far greater audience, but his comments on Whytt doomed the latter to obscurity as a disciple of Stahl. The occasional figure like Laycock (1848)[8] took up the essential difference between Whytt and Stahl—Whytt's concept of the unconscious mind—and employed it in psychiatry. Such attitudes were isolated.

Cullen (1777)[9] and his contemporaries at Edinburgh were 'orthodox against materialism', yet their physiology needed to ask nothing of significance of the soul. This was in some ways in direct line from Whytt, who was highly respected: he had shown 'great strength of argument' in his considerations of the soul; he was 'the

[7] A. von Haller, *Elementa Physiologiae*, vol. 4, p. 394.
[8] R. Hunter and I. MacAlpine, op. cit., p. 1079.
[9] W. Cullen, *Institutions of Medicine*, Edinburgh, 1777. The date 1677 appears erroneously on the title page.

proper authority to be consulted'[10] in preference to Stahl and the mechanists. From notes taken from his lectures in 1772[11] it appears that Cullen, like Whytt, was anxious to explain what *does* happen in body-soul relationships rather than *how* it happens: whatever the conclusions, 'we must keep to the *language* of Whytt . . .'.

Yet Cullen could not agree with Whytt's coextension—the soul is seated in the brain and only there is capable of sensation 'and not in the sentient extremities'.[12] Other points over which Cullen disagreed with Whytt include the latter's observation that there can be no excessive intensity of nervous power in pathological cases. He speaks favourably of Whytt's notion that the specific sensitivity of nerves may alter in disease but is most impressed with what have here been called the 'laws of union' and quotes largely from Whytt. As for Whytt's work on nervous diseases, it has been said[13] that the term 'neurosis', introduced in Cullen's scheme of classification of diseases, is heir to some of Whytt's ideas.

A later Edinburgh professor, W. P. Alison,[14] observed that Whytt, Stahl and Cullen all conceived erroneous notions of the functions of the nervous system, yet favoured Whytt's account of sympathetic actions controlled by a centralized sentient principle in preference to explanations involving connections near to the origins of the nerves. We have seen how Johnstone (whose publications continued at least until 1770) had a just idea of Whytt's work, as had two figures of the later history of the reflex, Unzer and Prochaska.[15]

These latter two, however, were research workers following up the literature of their subject, and in the specialized field of the reflex action, some knowledge of Whytt's work was kept alive by Marshall Hall (1850),[16] Brown-Séquard (1858)[17] and Seller (1862). Apart from this, historical opinion soon reverted to placing Whytt among the Stahlians. Early works of reference, like the historical medical dictionary of Dezeimeris (1839) and the *Biographie Universelle* of 1843 do so, and begin a tradition which has lasted up to the modern histories of medicine, of which Garrison's book of 1929[18] is but a single example.

[10] W. Cullen, *Works*, Edinburgh, 1827, vol. 1, p. 19.
[11] Quoted by W. Wightman, 'Wars of Ideas in Neurological Science', *The History and Philosophy of Knowledge of the Brain and its Functions*, ed. F. N. L. Poynter, Oxford, 1958, p. 134.
[12] W. Cullen, *Works*, p. 26.
[13] R. Hunter and I. MacAlpine, op. cit., p. 473.
[14] W. P. Alison, *Outlines of Physiology and Pathology*, Edinburgh, 1833, pp. viii, 266, 269.
[15] G. Canguilhem, op. cit., p. 109.
[16] Sir G. Jefferson, op. cit., p. 309.
[17] W. Seller, op. cit.
[18] F. H. Garrison, op. cit., p. 312.

To call Whytt a Stahlian is one cause of his undeserved obscurity. Perhaps others may be his early death or the jealousy of a colleague. However, we shall be on firmer ground if we examine the nature of his contribution to medicine. The concept of the reflex is not a simple one, and the several histories of it show that it took more than a century to reach anything like its final form. The precise significance of Whytt's contribution could not have been grasped until it could be seen in this perspective, from some distance. To Whytt, his contemporaries and those who came a little later, but most particularly to Whytt, what we understand by 'reflex' was a part of the wider phenomenon of sympathy. The threads of the as yet unwritten history of the sympathetic nervous system are still confused about Whytt's part in the development of neurophysiology.

Thus earlier accounts of his work concentrate on his analysis and treatment of nervous diseases at the expense of his consideration of animal motions, and so his name became associated with a subject of less interest for later historians, for whom, meanwhile, the developing idea of the reflex invited inspection.

In this way practitioners of the late eighteenth century may have used Whytt's book on nervous diseases as an authority (as William Perfect[19] did) and its influence certainly eclipsed that of the essay on animal motions. James Adair (1786) observed:

Upwards of thirty years ago, a treatise on nervous diseases was published by my quondam, learned and ingenious perceptor, Dr. Whytt, Professor of Physick, at Edinburgh. Before the publication of this book, people of fashion had not the least idea that they had nerves; but a fashionable apothecary of my acquaintance, having cast his eye over the book, and having often been puzzled by the enquiries of his patients concerning the nature and causes of their complaints, derived from thence a hint, by which he cut the gordian knot—'*Madam, you are nervous*'; the solution was quite satisfactory, the term became fashionable, and spleen, vapours and hyp, were forgotten.[20]

Adair's fashionable apothecary friend was not alone in seeing the advantages of Whytt's treatment of nervous diseases. The second half of William Smith's *A Dissertation on the Nerves* reads like a condensed and popularized (and largely unacknowledged) restatement of Whytt's discussion. He does, however, mention Whytt by name in recommending several of the latter's remedies,[21] and

[19] R. Hunter and I. MacAlpine, op. cit., p. 501.
[20] Ibid., p. 490.
[21] W. Smith, *A Dissertation on the Nerves*, London, 1768, pp. 199, 201, 211, 212, 231, 234, 236, 243.

occasionally owns a debt to Cheyne. The third author he seems to draw from is Nicholas Robinson,[22] whence come the *machinulae* and the animal aether of the nerves, which together provide a purely mechanical scheme of sensation and motion.

Even in this, Smith is not as original as he would wish to appear, and several passages in the first part of the book (where he deals with the motions of animals) are taken directly and without acknowledgement from Whytt's essay on the vital and involuntary motions. One such passage is Whytt's comparison of the Cartesian animal automata to 'so many curious pieces of clockwork wound up and set a going'.[23]

Smith's physiology is in fact that of Whytt with the important difference that the soul is limited spatially and functionally to the sensorium at the termination of the nerves. This soul is like Haller's, providing no more than consciousness, the origin of voluntary motion. Man, says Smith, lives on three levels: purely mechanical 'powers of vegetation' perform the vital and involuntary motions, 'animal' life is the source of voluntary actions, and in addition man has a spiritual existence. The vital motions come about like those described by Whytt, with stimulus and response, but without the intervening sentient principle. The oscillations of the small blood vessels; the automatically 'wise' involuntary actions which may yet endanger the fabric of the body; the necessary and proportional relation between stimulus and response, so that all vital motions are performed equally well by 'infants, ideots and brutes'; the movement of food in the gut, blood in the heart and air in the lungs; the details of the change of circulation of the foetus at birth; the action of opium on the nerves, and, lastly, the passage 'for the nerves of different organs are so constituted as to be very differently affected, even by the same things'[24] are all taken verbatim or very little changed, and unacknowledged, from Whytt. They include several important physiological ideas which seem to have got into the general medical literature in this kind of way, while his ideas on the soul were forgotten in the manner we have discussed above.

The only acknowledgement that Smith makes, indeed, to Whytt is just over this point of the soul. Smith is at considerable pains to prove its immateriality and quotes from Whytt to support his

---

[22] N. Robinson, *A New System of the Spleen, Vapours and Hypochondriack Melancholy*, London, 1729.

[23] This phrase seems to have become popular. It caught the attention of the reviewer in the *Monthly Review* (see p. 9) and is noted by several readers of Whytt's book.

[24] W. Smith, op. cit., p. 93. (From Whytt's *Works*, p. 29).

argument. He then observes that Whytt 'has been accused of materialism, and indeed I cannot vindicate his doctrine from these unhappy conclusions, though I verily believe he did not see them.' These 'unhappy conclusions' of materiality are criticisms which follow from Whytt's doctrine of the extension of the soul: his opponents argued that this and its 'divisibility' were properties of matter. Because of these difficulties Smith left the soul out of his physiological speculations, yet with others coming after Whytt, he adopted the remainder of his physiology.

Appendix

AN INVENTORY OF THE RIGHTS OF THE LANDS OF BENNOCHY RAMBROG AND EIGHTY ACRES OF LANDS OF ABBOTSHALL BELONGING TO ROBERT WHYTT ESQ. 1768 ELDEST SON OF THE DECEASED DR. ROBERT WHYTT OF BENNOCHY.[1].

1. Charter by William Earl of Dalhousie and George, Lord Ramsay, his son with consent of Dame Anna Heeming, his spouse in favour of Margaret Duray relict of George Burvy Burgess of Kirkcaldy and George Christian Agnes and Alison Burvies his children of an @rent of 240 marks furth of the lands of Abbotshall dated 11th & 14th March 1653.

2. Sasine in favour of the said Margaret Duray and of the said George Christian Agnes and Alison Burvies her children upon the penny charter 18 May 1653.

3. Charter by William Earl of Dalhousie, Lord Ramsay of Carrington his son. With consent of Dame Anna Heeming his spouse in favour of Robert Whytt and Janet Tennant his spouse and others of certain @rent and particularly of an @rent of £120 but liftable furth of the lands of Abbotshall dated 11 and 14th. March 1653.

4. Charter by William Earl of Dalhousie, Lord Ramsay of Carrington and George Lord Ramsay his son, in favour of Isabel Dwice relict of deceased James Whyte skipper. . . . of Kirkcaldy and Thomas and John Whyte his children of @rent of 480 marks. . . . to the sum of 8000 marks furth of the lands of Abbotshall dated 11th and 14th. March 1653.

5. Sasine in favour of the said Isabel Duray and her said children of the said @rents furth of the said lands of Abbotshall dated 18th. May 1653 and registered in the particular register of sasines at Coupar 13th. June 1653.

6. Charter by William Earl of Dalhousie Lord Ramsay of Carrington George Ramsay his son in favour of John Williamson elder Burgess of Kirkcaldy Janet Balcanquil relict of William Williamson Burgess . . . his brother Catherine Lundy . . . . . William McGuilder and Geo. Mike Mariner there of several @rents furth

---

[1] This copy of an earlier list is among the papers of E. W. M. Balfour Melville, now in the Scottish Record Office.

of the lands of the lands of Abbotshall Milnland . . . . etc. except the lands of Sharess dated 11th and 14th. March 1653.

7. Sasine upon the said charter in favour of the said Jo. Williamson Janet Balcanquil, Catherine Lundy and Geo. Mike of the said 3 @rents furth of the lands of Abbotshall dated 18th. May 1653 and registered in the particular register at Coupar 30th. June 1653.

8. Charter by William Earl of Dalhousie Lord Ramsay of Carrington George Lord Ramsay his son with consent of Dame Anna Heeming his spouse in favour of Mr Frederick Carmichael Minister at Auchterdurnay of a @rent of £42/8/– to the said Mr Frederick Carmichael and £40 Scots to Mr John Chalmer with the lands and Barony of Abbotshall dated 28 April 1653.

9. Sasine upon the said charter in favour of the said Mr Frederick Carmichael John Chalmer of the said @rents furth of the lands Abbotshall dated 18 May 1653 and registered in the register of Sasines for the shire of Fife and Coupar 2nd. June 1653.

10. Sasine in favour of Robert Whytt and Janet Tennant his spouse, Agnes Bogher mother Thomas Wilson and John Bird of several @rents further of the lands of Abbotshall dated May 18th 1653. Registered in the Register of Sasines for the shire of Fife 30 June 1653.

11. Charter from Oliver Cromwell Protector, in favour of John Boswell in Glasness and his spouse of the land of Abbotshall and other. . . . from the Earl of Dalhousie dated 17 June 1654.

12. Sasine in the aforesaid charter in favour of John Boswell in the aforesaid lands dated 2nd. March 1654 registered in the particular register for Fifeshire 2nd. May 1654.

13. Charter in favour of Robert Whytt burgess of Kirkcaldy, Janet Tennant his spouse and John Whytt his eldest lawful son of the lands of . . . . 80 acres of lands of Abbotshall and teinds and appurtenance thereof granted by George Lord Ramsay with consent of Dame Anna Heeming his spouse dated 1654.

14. Sasine upon the said charter in favour of the said Robert Whytt and Janet Tennant his wife and John Whytt his son, of the said lands of Abbotshall and teinds and appurtenances thereof dated 17 July 1654 and registered in the particular register at Kirkcaldy 10th. August 1654.

15. Sasine in favour of Robert Whytt late bailey and burgess of Kirkcaldy of several @rents therein mentioned furth of the lands of Abbotshall dated 17 July 1654. Registered 147 on the register of Sasines for Fifeshire and Kirkcaldy 10 August 1654 (proceeding on the precept of sasine contained in disposition to him by John Williamson burgess of Kirkcaldy and a number of other persons therein named who had right. . . . . .)

170

16. Sasine in favour of Henry Lundel . . . . . and an @rent of £200 Scots furth of the lands of Bennochy dated 26 April 1656 upon a band or obligation by Sir John Wemyss of Bogie to him. Registered in the general register at Edinburgh dated 23rd June 1656.

18. Notorial copy of precept directed to the Keeper of the Privy Seal for a charter in favour of Sir Andrew Ramsay of the lands of Abbotshall and West Milne of Kirkcaldy dated 3rd December 1658. Attested 5 Sep. 1659.

19. Disposition by Sir John Wemyss of Bogie in favour of Robert Whytt of Purnie provost of the Burgh of Kirkcaldy of the lands of Rambrog dated 1st. June 1659.

20. Extract disposition by George Lord Ramsay and Dame Anna Heeming his spouse in favour of Robert Whytt Burgess of Kirkcaldy and Janet Tennant his wife in life rent and John Whytt   by way of   betwixt them their eldest son in fee of   acres of the lands of Abbotshall dated the   day of and registered in the book of council and session the 4th day of September 1662.

22. Horning and poin. . . . Robert Whytt and. . . . . Geo. Lord Ramsay dated 4th. and signed 7th. Sep. 1665.

23. Suspension. Geo. Lord Ramsay ag. Rob. Whytt Burgess of Kirkcaldy and spouse and son dated 28th. Sept. signeted 14th. Oct. 1665.

20. Instrument of Sasine in favour of Robert Whytt and Janet Tennant his wife of the lands of Rambrog dated 3 June 1659. Proceeding on. . . . . disposition from Sir John Wemyss of Bogie dated 1 June 1659.

24. Charter of confirmation under the great seal in favour of John Whytt only lawful son of Rob. Whytt of the lands of Rambrog dated 22 Feb. 1667.

25. Sasine in favour of James Melville brother german to Lord Geo. Melville of an @rent of 328 merks four shillings Scots furth of the lands of Bogie and Bennochy and others belonging to Sir John James Wemyss of Bogie date 31 Dec. 1670 and 4 Jan. 1671 and registered in the register of Sasines for ye shire of Fife 24 Jan. 1761 on an heritable bond granted by the said Sir John and Sir James Wemyss.

26. Extract disposition and assignation by Sir John Wemyss of Bogie with consent of Dame Elizabeth Eden his spouse and James Wemyss suar of Balthug in favour of John Whytt of the town and lands of Bennochy dated the 9th (and 27 and 28 June) 1671 and registered in the books of council and session 20th. Jan. 1700.

27. Copy of ditto.

28. Obs decreet of transumpt of the rights of the lands of

Abbotshall. Note. Part of it is torn away at the beginning so that the
. . . . . . do not appear but it is presumable it was obtained before
the Sherriff of Fife and dated sometime between 1650 and 1700.

29. Decree of trans. . . . . Before the Provost and Baileys of
Kirkcaldy of the rights of the lands of Bennochy Rambrog and
Smeetown etc in favour of John Whytt of Bennochy for a defence
of his rights to the lands of Bennochy and Rambrog purchased by
him from the said Sir John Wemyss dated 29 July 1671.

30. Instrument of resignation in the hands of the Barons of the
Exchequer in favour of John Whyte of Powran of the town and
lands of Bennochy dated 30 June 1671 proceeding on the priory
contained in the said disposition of Sir John Wemyss of Bogie to
time dated 27 and 28th. June 1671.

31. Charter of Resignation under the great seal in favour of
John Whytt of the lands and town of Bennochy dated 14 July 1671
proceeding on the resignation of Sir John Wemyss of Bogie.

32. Precept of Sasine under the Quarter Seal in favour of John
Whytt of Persin Burgess of Kirkcaldy for incesting him in the
lands of Bennochy dated 14 July 1671.

33. Sasine upon a precept of sasine 2nd. charter resignation of
the town and lands of Bennochy in favour of John Whytt dated
8th. August 1671 and registered in the register of Sasines for the
shire of Fife at Coupar 17 August 1671.

34. Sasine in favour of John Whytt of Bennochy of an @rent
of £200 Scots upliftable furth of the lands of Bennochy and kinds
(teinds) thereof and others dated 15 Jan. 1672 and registered in the
register of Sasines for the shire of Fife at Coupar 1st. Feb. 1672
proceeding in the precept of sasine continued in a disposition by
the said Henry Landel tenant in main at Bogie to the said John
Whytt.

35. General retour in favour of John Whytt as heir to Robert
Whytt his father dated 28 Feb. 1674.
Disposition and Assignation of Abbotshall and Sir Andrew Ramsay
of Waughton his eldest son and their ladies to John Whytt of
Bennochy of all right and title they had to the teinds parsonage
and vicarage of the said 80 acres of the lands of Abbotshall dated
10th and 24 Oct. 1676.

37. Copy discharge by John Whytt of Bennochy to Wm. Earl of
Dalhousie for what bonds he had upon his land. . . . . they being all
paid by the land got by his father from the Earl of Dalhousie dated
22nd June 1678.

16. (sic) Registered Charter by George Lord Ramsay with consent
of Dame Anna Heeming his spouse in implement of a contract at
minute of sale in favour of John Whytt and his spouse of these

80 acres of the lands of Abbotshall dated blank of 1654 and registered in the book of Session 24 June 1713.

38. Copy of an interlocitur pronounced by a committee of commissioners of supply met a Coupar on a petition given in by Bennochy @rent the revaluation of his glebe dated 21st. Aug. 1690.

39. Contract of marriage between Mr. Rob. Whytt of Bennochy and Miss Jean Murray daughter of the deceased Dr Anthony Murray of Woodend dated 16th. Feb. 1697.

40. Special retour of Rob. Whytt of Bennochy as heir to John Whytt of Bennochy his father in the lands of Bennochy Rambrog and Abbotshall dated 15th. Oct. 1697.

41. Extract service Robert Whytt of Bennochy as heir to John Whytt his father before the bailles of the Regality town of Dunfermaling. Dated 15th. Oct. 1697.

42. Sasine upon a precept furth of the chancery in favour of Robert Whytt of Bennochy as heir to John Whytt of Bennochy of the town and lands of Bennochy with the pertenance dated 27 Oct. 1697 and registered in the register of sasine for the shire of Fife at Coupar 8 Dec. 1697.

43. Sasine upon a precept furth of the chancery in favour of Rob. Whytt as heir to John Whytt of the town and lands Rambrog with pertenance dated 27 Oct. 1697 and registered in the Sherriff's court of Fife 8 Dec. 1697.

44. Sasines upon a precept furth of the said blank acres and blank paws of the lands of Abbotshall in favour of the said Rob. Whytt dated 28 Oct. 1697 and registered in the register of the sasines for Fifeshire 8 Dec. 1697. Upon a precept from ye Chancery directed to Sir Andrew Ramsay of Abbotshall the superior.

45. Extract decreed before the justices of the peace of the shire of Fife in the instance of Robert Whytt of Bennochy of John Wemyss of Bogie @rent straightening his park dykes dated 16 Aug. 1699.

46. Revocation by Rob. Whytt of Bennochy in favour of the heirs female of his body of a clause in favour of his heirs male contained in the contract of marriage dated 1st. Sep. 1704.

47. Principal summons of declaration at the instance of Mr Rob. Whytt of Bennochy advocate against Sir Andrew Ramsay elder of Abbotshall and Sir Andrew Ramsay younger of Waughton signed 22nd. Feb. 1705. Anon which decreet in absence is pronounced by Lord Fountainhall ordinary 18th. July 1706 Execution of said summons on paper apart.

48. Inhibition and Arrestment on said dependence dated 26 signeyed 27 Feb. 1705 with 2 executions on papers apart decreet sight still be extracted on this summons if that should at any time be judged necessary.

49. Precept of a clause constat of the 80 acres of land of Abbotshall and teinds thereof by Mr Andrew Ramsay in favour of Mr Rob. Whytt of Bennochy as heir to John Whytt of his father dated 7th. Sep. 1713.

50. Sasine of the said 80 acres and blank falls of the lands of Abbotshall and teinds in favour of Rob. Whytt of Bennochy upon the said precept of clare constat Mr Andrew Ramsay of Abbotshall to him as heir to John Whytt his father dated 8 Sep. 1713 registered in the Sheriff council books of the Shire of Fife at Coupar 14 Oct. 1713. The only reason that . . . .

51. Special retour in favours of George Whytt of Bennochy as heir to Rob. Whytt his father in the said lands of Bennochy Ramsay and acres in the lands of Abbotshall dated 29 April 1715.

52. Precept furth of the Chancery directed to the Bailey of the Regality of Dunfermaling for the intestine Geo. Whytt as heir to Rob. Whytt his father in the lands of Bennochy Rambrog dated 12 May 1715.

53. Precept furth of the Chancery directed to Mr Andrew Ramsay of Abbotshall superior for entering Geo. Whytt heir to Rob. Whytt his father in the said blank acres of land of Abbotshall dated 12 May 1715.

54. Instrument of Sasine on a precept furth of a Chancery of the lands of Bennochy and Rambrog in favour of Geo. Whytt of Bennochy as heir to Rob. Whytt his father dated 14 May 1715 registered in general register of sasine at Edinburgh 10 June 1715.

55. Instrument of Sasine in favour of Geo. Whytt of Bennochy of the said blank arces of the lands of Abbotshall dated 14 May 1715 and registered in the general register at Edinburgh 16 June 1715 proceeding on a precept furth of Chancery directed to Mr Andrew Ramsay the superior, note it appears that this saine not given by Mr. Andrew Ramsay on his bailey but by his bailey of the Regality of Dunfermiling.

56. Special retourn of the service of Dr Robert Whytt of Bennochy as heir to George Whytt of Bennochy his brother in the lands of Bennochy and Rambrog dated 2nd. June 1732.

57. Precept of clare constat of John Arnot of Arnot Baronet in favour of the said Dr Robert Whytt of Bennochy as heir to the said George Whytt his brother in the aforesaid 80 acres of land Arnot formerly Abbotshall with the teinds sheaves and purtenance dated 8 June 1732.

58. Precept furth of Chancery upon the said retour in favour of the said Dr Rob. Whytt for investing him on the said lands of Bennochy and Rambrog dated 13 June 1732.

59. Instrument of Sasine upon the said precept of clare constat

on the said 80 acres of the land of Arnot formerly Abbotshall in favour of the said Dr Robert Whytt dated 1st July 1732 and registered in the particular register of the saines for the Shire of Fife at Coupar 12 July same year.

60. Instrument of sasine in favour of the said Robert Whytt of the lands of Bennochy and Rambrog and apurtenance proceeding on said precept furth of the Chancery dated 1. July 1732 registered in the said particular register of 4th July 1732.

61. Memorandum as to the state of the teinds of the 80 acres of lands of Abbotshall belonging to Dr Robert Whytt of Bennochy dated 1743 (note in margin) principle disposition by the said George Whytt to the said Dr Robert Whytt of the said lands of Bennochy and Rambrog of the 80 acres of Abbotshall dated 18th. Aug. 1724. This disposition. . . . . . . it was thought proper to pass by as the Doctor made up his teinds on a service as appear . . . .

62. Discharge from Mr Alex. Murdocairay to Mr Robert Whytt of Bennochy of all that he could ask . . . .

63. Bond and obligation by Mr Alex Melville of Murdocairay to Mr Andrew Melville Doctor of Medicine for twenty thousand marks dated 17th. March 1702.

64. Bond of relief by Beatrice Linklater relict of deceased James Whytt skipper in Kirkcaldy to Robert Whytt of Bennochy dated 27th. Oct. 1703.

64. Obligation by Mr Andrew Aitken at the West Bridge of Endirwilr to Mr Robert Whytt of Bennochy dated 12 June 1700.

66. Bond of relief by George Earl of Melville to Robert Whytt of Bennochy 22 Jan. 1703.

67. Bond of relief by George Earl of Melville to David Earl of Leven to Robert Whytt of Bennochy dated 8th Dec. 1704.

68. Bond of relief John Whytt merchant . . . . . bailiff Kirkcaldy to Robert Whytt of Bennochy dated 28 May 1715.

69. Contract of marriage between Mr John Ramsay merchant in Edinburgh and Mrs Jean Whytt eldest daughter of deceased Mr Robert Whytt of Bennochy advocate dated 4th Sep. 1717.

70. Obligation by John Ramsay of Old Woodston and Andrew Ramsay of Abbotshall in favour of Mrs Jean Whytt eldest lawful daughter of deceased Mr Robert Whytt of Bennochy advocate dated 4th. Sep. 1717.

71. Contract of marriage between the Rev. Andrew Melville Minister of Melville of the Gospel at Monymead and Mrs Helen Whytt lawful daughter of Mr Robert Whytt of Bennochy advocate dated 17th. Sep. 1719.

72. Discharge by John Melville of Murdocairay son of the deceased Mr Alex. Melville of Murdocairay to the representative

of the deceased Mr Robert Whytt and Andrew Melville Dr. of medicine, they being tutors to him 18 July 1722.

73. Discharge and declaration by Mr Andrew Melville Dr. of Medicine to Walter Boswall of Balbarton and the heirs of Bennochy dated Feb 26th. 1725.

Diploma of the University of St. Andrews to Geo. Whytt of Bennochy to be a Doctor of Physic dated June 16th. 1726.

74. Discharge by Mr Andrew Melville Doctor of Med. to Lady Bennochy for £2/10/– sterling as a years rent of £50 from Candlemas 1724 to ditto 1725 due by her to him by bond without date.

INDEX

Adair, James, 166
Aetius, 27, 110
Albertus Magnus, 111, 114, 121
Albinus, Bernard, 4, 33, 38
Alcmaeon, 96, 97
Alfred of Sarashel (*The Englishman*), 112
Alison, W. P., 165
Alston, Charles, 3, 8, 9
  on lime water, 17–26
  on opium, 50–2
Anaxagoras, 97
Anaximenes, 95–7
Andreae, Tobias, 132
Anima, 104, 121, 125–6, 129, 132, 138, 155; see also *Animus* and Soul
Animist reaction to Descartes, 128, 139
Animus, 104, 121, 125–6, 155; see also *Anima* and Soul
Archeus, 128
Architas Tarentinus, 99
Argyll, *Duke of*, 8
Aristotle, 96–8, 104, 106–8, 152, 154
  influence in Middle Ages, 111–16, 120, 122, 128
  on soul, 100
Aristoxenus, 105
Armstrong, John, 3
Asclepiades, 85, 106, 107, 139, 145, 152
Astruc, Jean, 33, 90, 147
Athenaeus, 106
Atoms of soul, 97, 125, 133
Avicenna, 111, 112, 116

Back, Jacobus, 128, 139
Bacon, Francis, 86, 153
Baglivi, Georgius, 42, 59, 86, 88, 134, 139, 154
Balfour, *family*, 1
Balfour, James, 6
Balfour, John, 15
Balfour, Louisa, 6, 15
Balfour Melville, E. W. M., 1
Balgonie, *Lord*, 15
Barclay, Robert, 16
Bark, 49
Bartholin, Thomas, 123, 135
Bartholomew of England, 112
Bateman, *Lord*, 16
Battie, William, 144

Bauhin, Caspar, 32
Begue de Presle, Achille Le, 12
Behrens, R. A., 141, 147, 152, 162
Bell, *Sir* Charles, 40
Berangario da Carpi, 114
Berger, Johann Gottfried von, 52
Bernard, Claude, 59
Bernouille, John, 150
Biondo, 118, 119, 125
Black, Joseph, 17, 18, 20–6
Blisters, 48, 54
Boerhaave, Hermann, 4, 5, 9, 27, 39, 42, 62, 80, 81, 150, 151, 161
Bohn, Johannes, 85, 86
Bontekoe, Cornelius, 134
Borelli, Giovanni, 54, 55, 57, 61, 81
Borrich, Olaus, 52
Boyle, Robert, 39, 85–7, 145, 153
Brain
  and opium, 51
  and sympathy, 40, 41
  in nervous activity, 60
  ventricles of, 102, 109–16
  as seat of soul, 93–168
Bremond, François, 80
Brocklesby, Richard, 63, 67, 68
Browne, *Sir* Thomas, 127
Brown-Séquard, Charles Edouard, 165
Brydone, Patrick, 47
Buccaferrea, Ludovic, 122
Buccinum Ampullatum, 50
Buchanan, Elizabeth, 6, 8
Burggrav, J. Philipp, 36
Bussière, Paul, 88
Butter, William, 6, 26

Caldani, Leopold, 52, 74, 88, 89
Caldesi, J. Baptista, 86, 134
Calor, 107
Camerarius, Elias, 146
Campbell, John, 26
Capillaries, 54
Carbon dioxide; see Black, Joseph
Carlsbad waters, 25
Castell, Peter, 68
Cat, Claude Le, 63
Celsus, 27
Centrum ovale as seat of soul, 133, 135
Cesalpino, Andrea, 119

177

Reisch, G., 114
Respiration, 5, 53, 79, 93, 94
Retina, 39, 75, 84
Ridley, Humphrey, 86, 134, 150
Riolan, Jean, 32, 120, 121, 122
Riverius, Lazarus, 32
Robertson, *General*, 5
Robertson, Helen, 4
Robinson, Bryan, 56
Robinson, Nicholas, 167
Roux, Augustine, 6
Rutherford, John, 3, 8, 11, 12, 15
Rutty, John, 17–19, 25

St. Ambrose, 108
St. Andrews University, 2, 4
St. Augustine, 110, 118, 136
St. Jerome, 108
St. Joseph of Copertino, 106
St. Luke, 106
St. Matthew, 106
St. Remigius, 110
Saint Romain, G. B. De, 133
St. Salvator's College, 2
Schelhammer, Gunther, 133
Schlosser, J. Albert, 25
Schwenke, Thomas, 87
Seller, William, 1, 165
Senac, Pierre, 60, 82
Sennert, Daniel, 32, 123
Sensation, 71–5, 85, 93, 96
Sensibility, 63–76
Sensorium commune, 34, 42, 50, 85, 96,
   101, 112–13, 116, 119, 123,
   126, 128, 129, 132–9, 142–3,
   146–7, 150, 158
Sensus communis, 103, 111–18, 121, 122,
   133; and see *Sensorium
   commune*
Sentient principle, see Soul
Servetus, Michael, 123
Shock, 64, 74, 86, 89
Simplicius, 110
Sinclair, Andrew, 3, 7, 8
Smellie, William, 52
Smith, William, 166
Soap, 5, 17, 18, 23
Soranus, 106, 119
Soul, 7, 9, 17, 30, 31, 33–6, 42, 54,
   69, 71–2, 75, 77–8, 80–91
   seat of, 93–148
   in physiology, 149–168

Specific energies of nerves, 38–40, 82,
   90, 156
Spinal cord, 41, 71, 77–92, 134, 158,
   160
Spinoza, Benedictus de, 127, 145
Spiritus, 107, 110
Springfield, Gottlob, 25
Stahl, Georg, 9, 14, 35, 57, 63, 91,
   118, 129, 138–142, 147, 149,
   158, 163–5
Steno, Nicolaus, 74, 134, 150
Stephens, Joanna, 17, 18
Stoics, 80, 103, 104
Stomach
   its sympathies, 36, 39, 51
   its sensitivity, 72
   as seat of soul, 120
Stone of bladder, 5, 6, 10, 11, 17–26
Strato, 103
Stuart, Alexander, 36, 86, 90, 150
Stuart, John, 22
Sublimate; see Ulcers
Supprian, F. Leberecht, 162
Swammerdam, Jan, 84
Swedenborg, Emanuel, 134, 137
Swieten, Gerard Van, 46, 50, 51, 59,
   67
Sympathetic trunk, 32, 33
Sympathy, 11, 28, 30–45, 68, 70, 75,
   77–92, 133, 147, 149, 157,
   160–1, 166

Tabor, J., 137
Tertullian, 106, 110, 119, 125, 136
Thales, 95
Thébault, 54
Theophilus, 110
Theophrastus, 102
Thymos, 94, 99, 105
Tissot, S., 162
Tyson, Edward, 88

Ulcers, 46
Unzer, Johann August, 165
Uterus, its sympathies, 31, 32, 36,
   38, 40

Vagus nerve in sympathy, 32
   Galen's 'sixth pair', 40
   'eighth pair' of eighteenth century,
   43

181

55663